T0129339

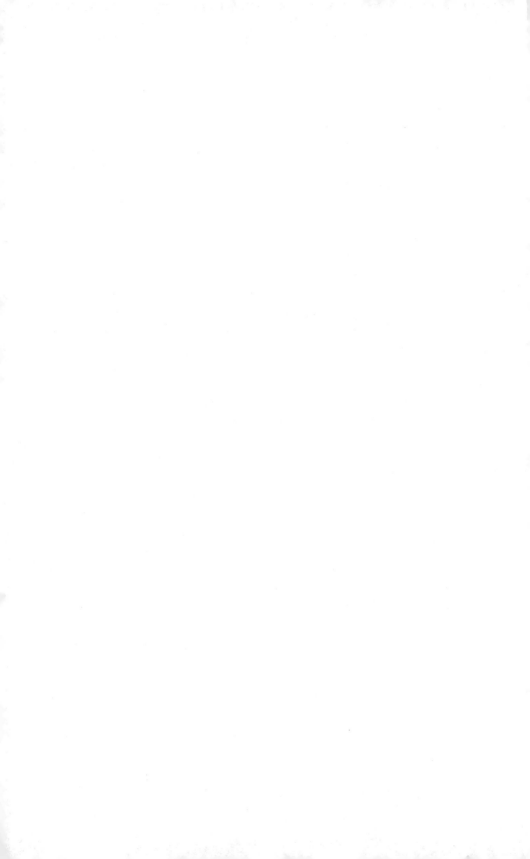

The PCOS
Mood Cure
Your Guide to Ending the Emotional Roller Coaster

Gretchen Kubacky, Psy.D.

The PCOS Psychologist

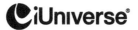

THE PCOS MOOD CURE
YOUR GUIDE TO ENDING THE EMOTIONAL ROLLER COASTER

The information, ideas, and suggestions in this book are not intended as a substitute for professional medical advice. Before following any suggestions contained in this book, you should consult your personal physician. Neither the author nor the publisher shall be liable or responsible for any loss or damage allegedly arising as a consequence of your use or application of any information or suggestions in this book.

iUniverse books may be ordered through booksellers or by contacting:

iUniverse
1663 Liberty Drive
Bloomington, IN 47403
www.iuniverse.com
1-800-Authors (1-800-288-4677)

Because of the dynamic nature of the Internet, any web addresses or links contained in this book may have changed since publication and may no longer be valid. The views expressed in this work are solely those of the author and do not necessarily reflect the views of the publisher, and the publisher hereby disclaims any responsibility for them.

Any people depicted in stock imagery provided by Getty Images are models, and such images are being used for illustrative purposes only.
Certain stock imagery © Getty Images.

ISBN: 978-1-5320-5217-0 (sc)
ISBN: 978-1-5320-5218-7 (e)

Library of Congress Control Number: 2018907954

Print information available on the last page.

iUniverse rev. date: 07/25/2018

To all the smart, strong, beautiful women who struggle with PCOS.

DISCLAIMER

This book is designed to provide information and coping mechanisms for the mental health issues related to Polycystic Ovary Syndrome (PCOS). It is sold with the understanding that the author is not providing medical, psychiatric, psychological, nutritional, or other professional advice or services.

If you have any physical or psychological condition that could be affected by the information provided in this book, you are encouraged to seek the advice of an appropriate medical or mental health professional before beginning or continuing any of the suggestions made from this book.

The purpose of this book is to educate, inspire, and encourage. The author shall have neither liability nor responsibility to any person or entity with respect to any loss or damage caused, or alleged to be caused, directly or indirectly, by the information contained in this book.

References made to patients are not references to specific people. Rather, they are composites of many people put together for the purposes of illustration and instruction. This was done to avoid revealing personally identifying information about any individual. Any resemblance to real persons, dead or alive, is purely coincidental.

CONTENTS

FOREWORD BY DR. SHEILA FORMAN

Polycystic Ovary Syndrome (PCOS) is a complex illness. For the millions of afflicted women, a "normal life" can seem out of reach. From mood swings and weight gain, to acne and infertility, PCOS wreaks havoc. With more than 200,000 women being diagnosed each year, PCOS patients need a healer – enter Dr. Gretchen Kubacky.

Dr. Kubacky is a compassionate health psychologist who has devoted her life to helping women cope with PCOS. A patient herself, Dr. Kubacky knows the heartache this diagnosis brings. Determined to end the suffering of as many women as possible, Dr. Kubacky has written this definitive guide to living well with PCOS.

Within these pages you, the PCOS patient, will find advice on dealing with the physical, psychological, and social consequences of this disease. With humor and wisdom, Dr. Kubacky shows you how to have a fuller, happier, and healthier life despite your diagnosis.

From *The PCOS Mood Cure* you will learn: what Polycystic Ovary Syndrome really is; why it is so hard to diagnose and treat and how PCOS affects your moods, weight, sleep and more. Using an integrative model, you will discover which medications and supplements could help you. You will come to understand the role food plays in your emotions and what you can do about it. And, maybe most importantly, you will be given a complete set of life skills including coping with emotions, dealing with chronic pain, improving sleep, and managing stress. Grounded in science and full of valuable resources, *The PCOS Mood Cure* is all you will need to feel better.

As a psychologist specializing in weight and eating issues, I understand the additional challenges faced by PCOS patients. I see the emotional toll that excess weight causes. I bear witness to the loss of self-esteem that facial hair and acne lead to. I calm the rollercoaster driven by mood swings. It's hard enough coming to terms with the pain and disappointments that life dishes out without having the extra burden of PCOS. I am so happy to finally have a book I can give to my patients to help them on their journey. With the insight and information from *The PCOS Mood Cure,* they feel more optimistic about their future. If you are working with a psychologist, I encourage you to give her a copy of this book. The more she knows, the more she can help you.

PCOS is a chronic condition that could rob you of a satisfying life, if it is not managed properly. The good news is that with the right support, PCOS does not have to stop you from having the life you want. You now have in your hands the best assistance you can ask for. With Dr. Kubacky as your guide, you can overcome the misery PCOS has bestowed upon you. You can lose weight, end mood swings, get good sleep, and build the loving relationships you long for.

So don't delay. Open the book, dig in, and let Dr. Kubacky show you the path to PCOS wellness.

Sheila H. Forman, Ph.D.
Clinical Psychologist and Mindful Eating Instructor
Author of *Do You Use Food to Cope?* and *The Best Diet Begins in Your Mind*
www.TameYourAppetite.com
Santa Monica, California
March 2018

PREFACE

Polycystic Ovary Syndrome (PCOS) is usually diagnosed after a woman has undergone years of infertility, weight struggles, mood swings, skin problems, and invasive tests. PCOS is currently estimated to affect as many as 22% of women. The need for psychological support is far greater than you might imagine – it's not just for the woman with PCOS, but for her family, friends, and co-workers who are also affected.

This book was borne out of my frustration as a PCOS patient experiencing innumerable symptoms, including depression, anxiety, mood swings, and an eating disorder, and finding almost no one who could help. This is what led me as a psychologist to specialize in working one-on-one with PCOS patients. I understand and empathize with what is lacking in patient care. This book is my attempt to provide that support and to change the dialogue about a disorder that affects roughly one in five women, from pre-puberty to post-menopause.

This book is a guide to managing the mental health, psychological, mood, and emotional issues related to PCOS. These issues cannot be managed effectively without addressing other lifestyle and well-being choices. Much of the information and suggestions contained herein can be useful in a do-it-yourself model of holistic health care. Further, it can also be of use to medical and psychological professionals, as well as friends and family.

The content provided is based on my knowledge and experience, which has evolved from operating in a void around PCOS psychology. It has developed through my unique lens and experience, not just what exists in the research. There is relatively little research on PCOS, particularly the psychological aspects. I have had to experiment and extrapolate from what is available, and my treatment approach is a work-in-progress. I could spend years updating and editing this book, but the need for it is so compelling at this time that I had to release it NOW. I hope the book will galvanize further research into the complexities of PCOS-related psychological conditions.

How to Use This Book

This book is designed as a lifestyle guide. You can read it cover to cover, or pick and choose the pieces you're most eager to address immediately. There is a comprehensive overview of the most common mental health issues affecting PCOS patients, including depression, anxiety, mood swings, irritability, eating disorders, and sleep problems. I also briefly address chronic pain issues, sexual health, infertility, and relationship issues that PCOS patients face.

Each chapter is a self-contained discussion on an individual topic, but several issues span categories and are cross-referenced. For example, you can jump straight to *Chapter 5: Insomnia and Other Sleep Disorders*, followed by *Chapter 17: Improving Sleep*, if you know sleep is your biggest problem. But you will derive the greatest benefit from the book if you read it all the way through, in the order written, and then use it later as a reference book, returning to specific chapters as needed.

If you are newly diagnosed and short on time, I suggest you read *Chapters 1, 2, and 3*, then *Chapter 12: Getting Proactive; Chapter 9: Food Essentials for Mental Health; Chapter 17: Improving Sleep*, and *Chapter 18: Exercising for Health*. This will give you a solid foundation for managing your PCOS.

Finally, I am aware that the idea of completely overhauling your lifestyle and ways of coping with PCOS is daunting. It can be expensive, time-consuming, and just plain difficult. So, decide what seems most useful right now, be patient with yourself, and return to the rest later. Whatever you can do now will undoubtedly be helpful. I hope you find the book useful, informative, actionable, and maybe even a little entertaining at times.

A Special Note for
Teens with PCOS

If you are a teenager with PCOS, then you might want to read this special introduction before anything else in the book. And, if you've already been flipping through the pages and seeing topics such as pregnancy, marriage, relationships, health complications and menopause, you might be wondering if this book is for you?

The answer is YES.

In fact, maybe it's especially for you! While it certainly may not seem like it now, finding out about your PCOS at an early age is actually an advantage. Yes, really! And one that many older women today didn't have. For the "pioneering" PCOS women who are now aged in their 50s and 60s, a diagnosis may have taken decades. Even then, there were few answers, with most of the medical community not understanding the questions. These women are now facing new frontiers – what does PCOS mean in menopause? Research takes time. Diabetes and pre-diabetes; thyroid, mood, hormone and metabolic disorders are all getting more research dollars, and more media attention. Eventually, some of this research will have meaningful implications for PCOS.

It's hard to set aside your impatience, I know, but answers are coming. Almost every day I read or hear something interesting that might have relevance, now or eventually, to the treatment and management of PCOS. And the lessons learned by the older PCOS pioneers are proving a great legacy for all the new generation of PCOS cysters, such as you.

One thing I would like to reassure you is that PCOS does get better if you get a grasp on it now and learn how to accept it. You can also use this time to identify your own problem areas and best coping skills and strategies. While understanding that PCOS is a chronic disease may be very frightening for you right now, acceptance is important on your road to good health.

Did you know that PCOS improves if you treat it well? It's like your annoying little sister who bugs you all the time. It wants attention – positive attention, and lots of it. If you can learn how to respect that and treat it well, life is sure going to become a lot easier.

Being a "digital native" is another advantage of your age. The internet is already your friend. Today, more than any time in history, advice is readily available for you to consume. The world has opened up in amazing ways; you just have to look. I'm sure you don't feel limited by the opening hours at the local library, or the lack of a car to get you there. Books on every topic imaginable can be found on Amazon – but I'll bet you probably aren't even fazed if you don't have any money to buy one. Much of what you need to know is available for free! You don't have to think twice about jumping on your smart phone or device to look up or download something. This is easy and natural for you; you can stay on top of 500 things all at once. Because you are probably still in school, you're getting educated about lots of other things right now – so you are used to studying, researching, reading, and assimilating. PCOS health care is just another aspect of education. Think how much harder it would be to start learning all of this from scratch later in life.

Because of your ability to identify friends, communities, and other like-minded individuals through social media, as well as in person, you will also have an easier time tracking down support groups, doctors, new research, and treatment options. You get that it's actually quite easy to ask a stranger for assistance. You already have faith that someone out there knows something that might help you. By reading this book, you're learning a lot about what cautions to take in considering these resources.

Knowledge is power (I tend to repeat that a lot!) – so make use of all your resources.

Your age advantage means you can track your labs and other health indicators over a long period of time. Again, this is about deriving power from knowledge. Having good baseline numbers from your teen years is the best way to know what's normal for you. It's not necessary to keep a lifetime of medical records, although of course you should always have some basic information about childhood immunizations and that sort of thing. But it's about knowing things like how travel affects your eating and exercise habits, what stress does to your lab work, and how different medications do or don't work for you.

I know that right now, like any other teenager, you're a little obsessed with how you look. Having PCOS-related physical issues – like acne or excess hair or weight – make this an even bigger deal. But, there are more and more solutions for these problems. Yes, they take time, money, and consistent application or effort, but they're often quite effective. Manufacturers are pouring millions of dollars into researching and producing more effective products, appliances, and treatments for acne, hair loss, and excess weight management. There's so much hope for the future!

There's also much less stigma about mental health issues now, and about the medications used to treat them. Antidepressants are readily available. Depression screenings happen at school and at work. Everyone talks about their anxiety. Doctors are more educated about the effect of mental health on physical health (not always, but they've got their learning curve too). Because of all this, you have a better chance of getting "caught" if you're falling into depression. This is a good thing.

Later on, you might even avoid infertility issues altogether by going into pregnancy planning with detailed knowledge of the potential difficulties and seeking help sooner rather than later. This will help you to deal with it more calmly and effectively. It won't be a panic or a surprise. It will still be a drag, but you'll know there are specific things you can do to address the problem.

As a teenager with PCOS you can develop good habits now, instead of waiting a decade – or two or three – when major damage has already been done.

By making it a habit to eat well, monitor your health, exercise and manage your stress, you will be far ahead of your peers when they start hitting their 40s and 50s and find that things are falling apart at an alarming rate. You'll be able to say, "been there, done that," and offer them hope and guidance, while you are secure in the knowledge that you know how to take care of your health, and have been doing so "forever."

So, by taking control of your PCOS now, you can save time, money and grief by managing your own medical life from this point forward (with appropriate parental supervision, of course). I absolutely recommend the rest of this book to you, even if it's addressing topics that don't seem relevant right now. PCOS is a lifetime condition, and it changes over time. But with good resources at your side, you will know what to look for. Absorb what information is useful for now – and save the rest for the future.

ACKNOWLEDGMENTS

No book would be complete without an acknowledgment of those individuals and organizations that have contributed significantly to its development and contents. I particularly wish to express my gratitude to the following:

Tabby Biddle, M.A.; Pejman Cohan, M.D.; Sheila Forman, J.D., Ph.D.; Steve Glass, Psy.D.; Angela Grassi, M.S., R.D., L.D.N.; Bruce Gregory, Ph.D.; Marki Knox, M.D.; Bonnie Modugno, M.S., R.D.; Lisa Moore, M.D.; Sam Najmabadi, M.D.; Sasha Ottey, M.S.; William Patterson; Nikole Peterson; Paula Shearer (Editor); Kimberly Smith; The Stone Center at Wellesley; Ryan Witherspoon, M.A.; Monika Woolsey, M.S., R.D.; Hillary Wright, M.Ed., R.D.N.; and Lidia Zylowska, M.D.

And finally, a big thank you to all my clients, listeners, friends, fans, and readers, whose PCOS stories have inspired me, saddened me, angered me, caused me to think and research and dig a little deeper, and galvanized me into writing this book so that I could offer a consolidated reference point for information on managing the emotional and psychological issues of PCOS.

I am grateful to have such an amazing, patient, brilliant, creative, and thoughtful professional and personal support group in my life, and for their contributions to the creation of this book.

To your health!

Gretchen Kubacky, Psy.D.
Health Psychologist
Founder of PCOS Wellness
Certified Bereavement Facilitator
www.DrGretchenKubacky.com
www.PCOSwellness.com
@AskDrGretchen

GRETCHEN'S STORY

I was diagnosed with Polycystic Ovarian Syndrome (PCOS) in my early 20s, by a doctor who didn't explain what I had, what my symptoms meant, how to manage the symptoms (other than birth control pills), or what this diagnosis meant for my long-term health and well-being. Thirty years later, have I got a story to tell!

I developed early and started to gain weight, especially abdominal fat, at the same time. I tried very hard to diet, starting when I was 10 years old, but it was nearly impossible to contain my cravings for carbohydrates. I felt ashamed and out of control because I was fatter than my friends, and I had no idea there might be a biological reason for my behavior. I just thought I was weak and lacked self-control, because that's what everyone kept telling me. My mom tried to bribe me into eating less. I desperately wanted to lose weight, so I could be "normal" and fit into the cute clothes other girls were able to wear. Health was irrelevant to me at that point; it was all about fitting in rather than standing out.

Throughout my entire adolescence, I subsisted on as little food as I could manage, and swam 200 laps per day. Sometimes, I would swim for five straight hours. Nowadays, I'd call that exercise bulimia (over-exercising in order to maintain or reduce weight), but I just thought it was a clever way to balance out what was going on in my body.

I got my period the month I turned 14, and it was irregular, which my family doctor said was normal. My periods were as short as three days or as long as 12 days, and they came as close together as two weeks or as far apart as several months. At one point, I didn't have a period for over one-and-a-half years. I didn't mind.

I wasn't able to exercise nearly as much in college, and I had also developed hypoglycemia (low blood sugar) which left me feeling weak, shaky, unfocused, and with difficulty concentrating. I was always hungry. I self-medicated with a steady supply of M&Ms. Needless to say, I gained even more weight. I hated my body, and was absolutely miserable in it, but tried to accept that I was just "big boned" and destined to be fat.

By the time I was 25, I felt so awful all the time that I ended up in an endocrinologist's office where I got a diagnosis of hypoglycemia and orders to lose weight. I think I weighed about 200 pounds at that time. I tried for a few months to stick to a very strict "well-balanced" diet that a registered dietician created for me, but I was constantly on the edge of hypoglycemia, or actually hypoglycemic. I was irritable all the time. I would get nervous, sweaty, have trembling hands and blurred vision, felt like I was starving, and be absolutely fixated on food almost every waking moment. It was not a good way to live, so I gave up trying and gained almost 70 pounds in one year. Sure, I was eating all the bad foods, but I was eating all the vegetables too, so I figured it was okay. No one told me that severe hypoglycemia is often a precursor to diabetes.

In addition to the excess weight, there was always the hair problem – a moustache and chin hairs that made me look a whole lot more like my grandmother than I wanted to look. I chalked it up to my German heritage, and kept on plucking, shaving, and waxing. I knew it wasn't quite normal, but I didn't think it was that abnormal either. Certainly, no doctor asked about it.

Two years later, I was diagnosed with early onset type 2 diabetes. I was scared, embarrassed, and ashamed. I believed I was the entire cause of my diabetes. And I knew better than to think that you just take a pill and then you don't have a diabetes problem.

PCOS was a side note while I dealt with the diabetes. I went on a rampage. I hadn't exercised consistently since I was a teenager, but fear drove me. I started with 10 minutes of walking and built up to walking more than an hour a day, and I focused on changing my diet. I persisted, and I lost 70 pounds. I managed my diabetes with only diet and exercise, my numbers were good, my doctors were enthralled and, oh yeah, I still had PCOS.

I had irregular Pap smears, with a lot of "atypical benign cells" and call-backs for repeat samplings, but none of my doctors suggested that I might have a bigger problem. In 1998, I had my first dilation and curettage (D&C) to remove these problem cells from my body, which turned out to be the first of nearly a dozen D&Cs during the next 14 years. I jokingly referred to it as my annual D&C. Along the way, I had so many punch biopsies that I thought my insides must be starting to look like Swiss cheese. I was trying to use humor, but the emotional side effects of these scary, painful, and inconvenient tests and treatments wore on me. I was tired of the pain, the expense, the anesthesia and painkillers and antibiotics and, of course, the threat of death (I've never signed a surgical consent form that didn't duly inform me of the risk of death).

I went on birth control pills, but still developed enlarged and painful cysts in my ovaries. Some of them kept growing and had to be removed surgically. Although there is a very small chance that a cyst could be cancerous, there's also a chance that a cyst could rupture and require emergency surgery, so I kept playing it safe and having the surgeries. I didn't know then that every surgery throws you into metabolic imbalance for six to 12 months. I kept having surgery after surgery.

In 2003, I added endometriosis and uterine polyps (and a subsequent couple of polypectomies) to my expanding list of gynecological diagnoses and procedures. I also added an excellent reproductive endocrinologist to my growing list of doctors, not realizing that I was referred to him because no one else actually knew what to do to "fix" me. My endocrinologists were jointly experimenting with various hormones in an attempt to rebalance my system. I'd buy a prescription, try it, have bad side effects, call the doctor, have another appointment, get another prescription, try it, have unacceptable side effects, and on and on and on. Again, I resorted to jokes – being a patient was my "hobby" – but I hated spending my life in a revolving door of medical appointments.

In 2004, I had a surgery-free year! My diabetes was under good control without medication, I was having semi-regular periods on birth control pills, and I dared to have a little hope that maybe my PCOS was contained. But I started off 2005 and every year thereafter for the next five years with a D&C. I never had to worry that I wouldn't meet my insurance deductible in a given year; I often met it within the first two weeks.

When I was 40 years old, I was finally in a relationship with someone who seemed like a good potential mate/father. We knew my age was an issue, and PCOS was an issue, but we figured we would try to get pregnant on our own anyway. We tried and failed for over a year. I felt the time pressure, but I still believed that there was a window of opportunity.

We were referred to a high-risk obstetrician/gynecologist. He ran down an extensive list of negatives: "advanced maternal age" and history of PCOS, diabetes, and hypothyroidism. His comment: "no one else in this town will touch you, and I don't recommend pregnancy, but if you proceed, I will take care of you" summed up my overall prognosis. He noted that I would be on a severely restricted diet, injectable insulin, and most likely complete hospitalization for the final trimester. Not bed rest. Hospitalization. I could not process all this bad news. When "maternal death" was mentioned as another potential complication, we immediately declared "game over."

Just as I was beginning to reassess my situation, I had developed another rapidly growing cyst, of an unidentified nature. I don't know about you, but when the doctor says: "I'm pretty sure it's not cancer, and it's not a baby, but I don't know what it is," it's kind of stressful! We scheduled surgery, and then a final check before surgery showed that things were looking even more complex, so the surgery was cancelled. My body seemed out of control.

A hysterectomy had been mentioned years before as a treatment possibility, but back then I wasn't interested. This time though, I was just outside the window of feasible fertility. My eggs had expired when I wasn't looking! I ended up making the difficult decision to have a partial hysterectomy.

I still wasn't willing to give up on finding a cure or at least a very good treatment for PCOS. My search led me to four gynecologists, four endocrinologists, a reproductive endocrinologist, 13 nutritionists, three naturopathic doctors, one classically-trained homeopath, 13 acupuncturists, and a functional medicine specialist to try to perfect a program.

I've had more lab tests than I could ever have imagined, diagnostic procedures I can't even pronounce let alone spell, and of course all the surgeries. I've tried Western pharmaceuticals of every permutation, homeopathy, colon hydrotherapy, abdominal massage, Chinese herbs, some extremely questionable Ayurvedic herbal preparations imported from India, and enough supplements to choke a horse – frequently up to 90 capsules per day, for months on end.

I also admit to trying everything from HCG (human chorionic gonadotropin) with a 500 calorie per day diet; no-carb, low-carb, very-low carb and the ketogenic diet; no wheat, no dairy, no caffeine, no alcohol, no sugar, no potential allergens, a vegetarian liver cleanse, multiple colon cleanses, the Paleo(lithic) diet, and a lot of elimination diets. I've tried most of the supplements and medications recommended for PCOS and/or diabetes. I've eaten too many calories, too few calories, the wrong calories, and done too much exercise, too little exercise, and the wrong exercise. In other words, I have been where you've been, done what you've done, and probably a whole lot more. I don't recommend it.

If a lot of this sounds out of control, it is – and it was. I'm not proud of it, because some of it was desperate and stupid and misguided. I've wasted phenomenal amounts of time, money, energy, and hope on promises of "the cure." But you do not have to experience everything I have experienced in my PCOS journey in order to improve your physical and emotional health.

Today, I practice all the self-care techniques that I am about to teach you. I try to remember to have fun with food, and that food is not the enemy. I try to remember that my body is not the enemy either. I acknowledge that my body has been through a lot and is deserving of great compassion and respect. Yours is too.

When I'm moody, irritable, or downright depressed, I see it as a signal to slow down and ask what healthy actions I need to take to help myself feel better. I'm a proactive patient who tracks her own numbers, does research, and continues to experiment with diet, exercise, and other self-care techniques. I also try to remain hopeful and optimistic about new developments in health care and PCOS research. I hope that my story and this book are inspirational and motivating for you.

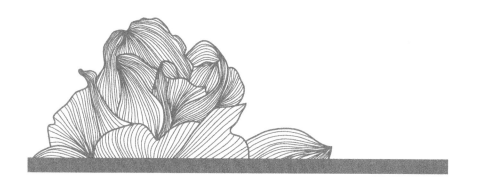

Part One:

What is PCOS?

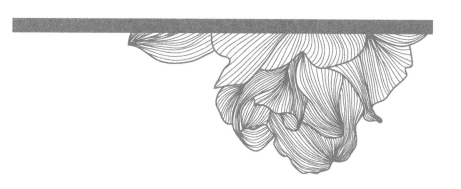

CHAPTER 1
What is PCOS?

Defining Polycystic Ovary Syndrome

PCOS, the most common endocrine disorder for women, is thought to occur due to a combination of genetic and environmental factors. These factors may include obesity, family history of PCOS or other endocrine disorders, exposure to environmental toxins, high levels of stress, or a history of trauma resulting in acute stress. Insulin resistance appears to be a predominant factor in PCOS as well.

Women with PCOS commonly experience:

- Menstrual irregularity
- Menstrual cramps
- Heavy menstrual bleeding
- Menstrual periods with clots
- Infertility
- Higher rates of miscarriage
- Difficulty breastfeeding
- Androgen excess
- Difficulty losing weight and staying at desired weight
- Abdominal fat
- Increased appetite
- Back pain
- Insulin resistance

- Cysts in their ovaries
- Higher risk factors for cardiovascular disease
- Pre-diabetes
- Early onset type 2 diabetes
- Non-alcoholic fatty liver disease
- Endometriosis
- High blood pressure
- High cholesterol
- Obstructive sleep apnea
- Fatigue
- Abdominal bloating
- Thyroid problems
- Male-pattern hair loss on the head
- Hirsutism (excess hair growth on the face and body)
- Acne on the face and body
- Skin tags
- Skin darkening (acanthosis nigricans)
- Hidradenitis suppurativa (painful pus-filled cysts)

Psychological symptoms include:

- Anxiety
- Depression
- Poor self-esteem
- Mood swings
- Irritability
- Brain fog
- Increased pain
- Fatigue
- Sleep problems
- Eating disorders
- High levels of frustration
- Embarrassment about physical appearance
- Feeling a lack of control over the situation/their bodies
- Worry

- Acute self-consciousness
- Fear of getting cancer
- Feeling different from others
- Loss of femininity
- Fearing for the future
- Losing control of one's temper easily
- Feeling tense
- Anger
- Tearfulness
- Isolation
- Feeling unattractive/unsexy
- Issues with libido
- Feeling suicidal

These symptom lists are extensive, yet incomplete, due to the complexity of the condition. The multi-systemic nature of the symptoms cause difficulty in obtaining diagnosis and treatment.

What PCOS is Not

PCOS is not the same as Premenstrual Syndrome (PMS), or Premenstrual Dysphoric Disorder (PMDD). However, many women with PCOS also experience PMS or PMDD. PCOS is not cancer, endometriosis, or infertility - although all those conditions can be caused or worsened by PCOS. Most importantly, PCOS is not "all in your head."

Diagnosing PCOS

In 2003, the Rotterdam European Society for Human Reproduction and the American Society of Reproductive Medicine sponsored a PCOS consensus workshop. They proposed that PCOS diagnosis included two of the following three criteria:

- Oligoovulation and/or anovulation (infrequent or lack of ovulation/menstruation)
- Clinical and/or biochemical hyperandrogenism
- Polycystic ovaries (as determined by ultrasound examination)

A medical examination for PCOS will typically assess menstrual patterns, obesity, insulin resistance, hirsutism, hair loss, and acne. Blood tests are utilized to measure hormone levels, glucose tolerance, fasting insulin levels, and related markers, such as C-reactive protein, a marker for inflammation.

What is the Treatment for PCOS?

PCOS unfortunately is usually treated in piecemeal fashion by numerous specialists who each address separate aspects of the patient's condition, with no single medical provider providing oversight or guidance. If PCOS were a broken bone, that type of approach might work. But the endocrine system is highly complex and requires a finely tuned balance in order to function optimally.

Lifestyle changes are the primary treatment recommendation for PCOS, with dietary management and increased exercise aimed at lowering insulin resistance and reducing weight. Other treatments focus on restoring/enhancing fertility, treating acne, reducing excess hair growth, restoring menstruation, and preventing or treating endometrial hyperplasia and cancer.

Standard treatment for decades has included birth control pills to help regulate periods, metformin (an insulin sensitizer) to reduce insulin resistance and prevent early onset type 2 diabetes, and spironolactone for hirsutism and acne. Assisted reproductive technology techniques and medications can help with achieving pregnancy. Dietary approaches have been variations of low-calorie diets and diabetes diets (designed to improve insulin resistance). Endometrial hyperplasia is sometimes treated with medication and sometimes with surgery. Problematic cysts may also be removed surgically.

Mental health issues, while common, are usually not addressed. Other than prescription medication, there are no unified treatment guidelines. Most medical doctors do not "prescribe" supplements, but there are a number that may be commonly recommended, including fish oil and Vitamin D. There is no PCOS-specific psychological treatment protocol for the mood, sleep, and eating disorders common in women with PCOS.

How Big is the PCOS Problem?

There is no cure for PCOS. This may be due, in part, to the fact that PCOS is one of the most poorly funded and researched health conditions despite the fact that it affects as many as 22% of women of all ages, races, and ethnicities. But diagnosis and awareness is improving, which means that numbers are likely to continue to rise. Given how little we really know about PCOS, it is hard to comprehensively define the scope of the problem, let alone develop effective treatment plans.

PCOS really only became part of the general women's health conversation perhaps a decade ago, although the condition first known as Stein-Leventhal Syndrome was "discovered" in 1935. I continue to regularly hear from women whose diagnosis was missed or delayed until very recently. I work one-on-one with women who have not been heard, have not received the treatment they needed when they needed it, and who have suffered needlessly.

When it comes to addressing mental health issues associated with PCOS – such as depression, mood swings, eating disorders, and insomnia – forget it: for decades, there has been no recommended psychological treatment. Again, I only began to connect the dots and delve further into treating patients with PCOS-associated mental health issues after I experienced profound depression and anxiety, infertility, a lifelong eating disorder, and all of the associated mood swings. This book is designed to save you from this emotional suffering, so you can live your healthiest and happiest life with PCOS.

CHAPTER 2

Why Living with PCOS is Hard

Just listing the predominant symptoms of obesity, mood swings, acne, hirsutism, and infertility should be enough to illustrate why living with PCOS is hard. You are constantly on a diet, but can never lose the weight; you cry over spilt milk (or over a TV commercial for deodorant); you are 40 but have the acne of a 14-year-old; or, you cannot make the dream of having children come true (and you don't know why).

But PCOS is also hard because, for the most part, it's an invisible disease. An astonishing number of medical professionals have never heard of it – they dismiss it, minimize it, or only know how to treat it with medication and surgery. The invisible (or mysterious) nature of the disease means that most people in your life just don't get why you're tired, cranky, and miserable most of the time. Friends, family, colleagues, and yes, even your doctors don't know that you have to try 10 times harder than anyone else with diet and exercise to show the slightest improvements. They just don't get it!

To add to the problem of diagnosing PCOS is the fact that it presents in several different ways too: not every PCOS patient is obese, for example. Once a diagnosis is given, then there are competing theories about causes and the best treatments, which are all based on a limited amount of research. Every day, PCOS has a negative effect on energy, mood, and brain processes that can lead to problems with school, work, sexuality, and relationships. And finally, there are the systemic and financial challenges: PCOS is expensive to treat, especially when you self-medicate with supplements that aren't covered by insurance, and many insurance plans don't cover fertility-related medications or procedures.

Why I Wrote This Book

PCOS affects not only the body, but also the brain. You just can't separate the two. Treatment of the psychological aspects of PCOS is essential to successfully treating the physical aspects of the syndrome. Managing eating disordered behavior, anxiety, brain fog, mood swings, irritability, and depression, as well as the elevated levels of stress that accompany PCOS are necessary for complete relief. My approach as a health psychologist is both holistic and integrative, because my experience is that anything less would be incomplete. In the end, most patients don't care how they get the desired results, but simply that they do achieve those results. This is therefore a very practical guide to taking charge of your PCOS and improving all aspects of your health.

How Will Health Psychology Help Me?

Naturopathic medicine utilizes the principle of Vis Medicatrix Naturae, translated as the healing power of nature. This principle suggests that the body has an inherent ability to establish, maintain, and restore health. The brain, being part of the body, also has a pull toward homeostasis. While I am not a naturopathic physician, I too believe that the body is designed to be self-healing, and that it requires proper support in order to do so. The more complex or long-standing the condition, the more support may be required. That support may take the form of traditional pharmaceuticals, nutritional support, supplements, bodywork, psychotherapy, support groups, education, and a variety of other resources and modalities that I will describe later.

As a health psychologist, I facilitate the process of healing both mind and body by helping patients identify the underlying causes and factors that may contribute to their illness(es) and their ability (or inability) to handle it effectively. These may include the syndrome itself, access to certain tests or specialists, lack of knowledge about diet and exercise (or incorrect information), a history of trauma, or the presence of other mental health issues. For women with PCOS, I teach coping and stress reduction skills, provide strategies for managing food cravings and mood swings, facilitate the grief process re: infertility and other losses, teach meditation and, most importantly, help them identify and use their own natural resources. I also teach them how to put together the best possible health care team and serve as their own advocate.

I do this by drawing on my resources, education, training, practical experience, ongoing study, and self-practice. I experiment on myself with the techniques I recommend here, such as yoga, meditation, and the use of certain behavior modification techniques. This book is an integration of my personal and clinical experience, professional and self-education, and multiple healing philosophies. It is a self-treatment plan that also reveals when it is better not to go it alone.

My goals for PCOS patients include increasing acceptance of their bodies, enhancing coping skills, improving life balance (which is so essential to achieving your best health with PCOS), and developing a personalized action plan that can be consistently implemented. I will teach you strategies to decrease the hyper-excitability of the brain, which is so characteristic of PCOS. This includes medical, nutritional, and psychological approaches such as meditation, hormonal regulation, dietary modifications, exercise, and other ways of decreasing inflammation. The net result is less stress, less irritability, less mood swings, less anxiety and depression - and more control over your present and future health.

The purpose of this book is multi-fold:

- First and foremost, it is to provide education and information about the specifics of PCOS and mental health. It integrates my personal experience as a PCOS patient with my professional experience as a health psychologist specializing in endocrine disorders and other chronic illnesses.

- It is designed to stimulate examination and use of your resources by offering some of my resources and thought processes to help you access your internal wisdom.

- Encouraging you to ask questions about your approach to your health, well-being, self-care, relationships and attitude.

- Offering hope that you can gain some measure of control over your PCOS.

- Providing encouragement by sharing case examples (integrated throughout) of other women who are making peace with PCOS and learning how to live a full and happy life with the diagnosis.

- Lending support in the form of sharing, concrete suggestions for action steps, and resources for making contact with other women with PCOS, professionals, and informed laypeople who understand and care about PCOS.

- Delivering a vision for successful lifetime self-management of PCOS.

CHAPTER 3

Hormones, Mood, and Stress

The Big Picture

It's no secret that hormones affect mood. Since PCOS is all about hormones, of course mood is going to be affected! PCOS has been described as "the perfect endocrine storm," and I'd say that's an apt description. The endocrine system is already a thing of remarkable and dramatic complexity, and when one part of it goes awry, there's a domino effect, and the rest of it follows. Pretty soon, everything is off-kilter - from your periods to your hair growth, the color and texture of your skin, and the basic functioning of your brain.

In order to properly treat your PCOS mood, it's important to have a clear picture of what's going on with you. Differentiating normal from abnormal moods can be extra challenging with PCOS. While there is a finite set of mental health diagnoses, the presentations are different from patient to patient. I'm always looking for the links and patterns between physical balance/imbalance and a woman's mood, depression, irritability, or other emotional or functional symptoms.

Many of us have tried anti-depressants or other prescription medications to help with the ups and downs of PCOS. Over-the-counter medications like Sam-E, Kava, and so on are also common self-prescriptions. To further complicate matters, we have varying diets, ethnicities, exercise habits, sleep statistics, and medications. Our moods and how medications work (or if they work at all, or for how long) are affected by a person's age, gender, body mass, ethnicity, and general state of health. In other words, if you put a petite 80-year-old Asian woman on an anti-depressant, and a 200 pound 23-year old African-American woman with PCOS on the same dose of medication, you'd probably be getting it wrong, yet that's how medications get dosed all the time. If you've felt like all of this is just a guessing game, there's some truth to that!

Understanding How Stress Affects Your Hormones

Despite all of these complications, it's really important to understand how stress affects your hormones. Firstly, you need to know simply that stress produces a hormonal response. Many of those responses are predictable, but many aren't. Our stress responses are the same as they were in ancient times, but these days, we're faced with an infinitely higher number of stressors. This leads to physical and emotional exhaustion and depletion.

Stress can be caused by any number of things, including most aspects of daily life - and even good or positive events, not just negative or scary events. Getting married, starting a new relationship, graduating from college, or losing 20 pounds can all produce stress, just like getting in a car accident, trying to make a deadline at work, or getting raped. But that doesn't mean you should stop doing the good things – just be aware that even positive stressors are still stressors. All those stress hormones, if left unmanaged, can cause disruptions to your endocrine system. When the endocrine system is already abnormal, as it is in PCOS, those stress effects tend to hit harder and earlier, and have more and longer-lasting negative effects.

The Good Kind of Stress

When you're stressed, a whole bunch of things happen inside your body. Your adrenal glands release adrenaline and cortisol, which give you an energy boost – you're ready to go! This "fight or flight" response is the body getting ready to take extreme physical action involving extra strength, speed and endurance. You're probably already familiar with the terms "adrenaline rush" or "adrenaline junkie," or you've heard about average people who can suddenly lift a car off a person who is trapped underneath.

When adrenaline is present, you experience:

- Increased heart rate, heart palpitations, sweating or anxiety.
- An increase in blood pressure.
- Rising blood sugar levels. Insulin increases to combat the rising blood sugar levels.
- Cold hands (a fear response).
- An inability to think clearly (this is about survival instinct, not refined thought).
- A pause in digestive processes (who needs digestion when you're about to get eaten by a wooly mammoth?).
- Increases in cortisol secretion.
- Decreases in progesterone.
- A rise in estrogen levels.

If you really are in immediate physical danger, these are all useful physical adaptations that allow you to fight back hard or run away. They're sending extra fuel to your muscles, shutting down unnecessary or distracting processes, and establishing a panic response that sends you into action.

The Bad Side of Stress

But if stress is a constant way of life, instead of an occasional event, excess exposure to hormones (primarily cortisol, adrenaline, and insulin) can be harmful, and you might end up with:

- A compromised immune system – you know how you always get sick right during those super-busy times at work?
- Problems with your thyroid.
- Irritability, being judgmental, and feeling on edge all the time.

- Tiredness, lethargy, lack of interest, and flat-out exhaustion.
- Cravings for sugar, bread, and other carbohydrates (the brain needs to replenish its glucose fuel supply which got expended during the stress event).
- Confused thinking.
- Weight gain.
- Decreased libido (sex drive).
- Abdominal bloating and/or abdominal weight gain (a response to excess cortisol).
- Breast discomfort.
- Acne, other rashes or flare-ups of skin conditions, such as eczema and psoriasis.
- Insomnia, which may further contribute to irritability and depression.

That sounds like the primary PCOS symptoms, in a nutshell, doesn't it? Now you understand why you're feeling the way you're feeling, especially if you're experiencing depression or anxiety. This is an ultra-simplified explanation, of course, but it's enough to give context to what goes on with PCOS-related psychological symptoms. You can see that hormones affect every aspect of our physical and mental wellbeing, and every system in the body. Note again that the endocrine system is complex, interacts with all the other systems of the body, and is a system with a very delicate balance that is easily upset. The good news is that small adjustments to your body chemistry may also bring the system back into line relatively quickly. In other cases, finding balance may require some hard work, thoughtfulness, and expert assistance.

PCOS Hormones

Testosterone is usually thought of as the male hormone. But in PCOS, testosterone and the other androgens are usually unbalanced. Testosterone has many vital roles in women and, like the other sex hormones, starts to decline with age. Many younger women who have been on birth control pills may also have low testosterone and experience symptoms associated with low testosterone levels. Symptoms associated with testosterone deficiency include increased submissiveness, rigidity, depressed drive and initiative, anxiety, poor memory, and low sex drive. In other words, problematic as it may be for a woman with PCOS, a little testosterone does keep you from feeling weak, wimpy, and unmotivated.

Estrogen and Progesterone are different hormones, but they work in conjunction with one another. As with testosterone, estrogen and progesterone decline with age, but at what age is unique to each woman, and the decline may not happen until as late as menopause. It could happen much earlier (or pretty much whenever it pleases, is what it can feel like with PCOS), and/or have varying highs and lows throughout a woman's lifetime. You may have heard, for example, that too much fat means you are estrogen dominant – and yet you have mood symptoms associated with estrogen deficiency! Reproductive status, other hormones, medications, stressors, and diet affect these levels as well.

Some of the mood-related symptoms can include depression and lack of sex drive. Tiredness and memory issues are also potential problems related to estrogen deficiency. Excess estrogen or progesterone deficiency may cause more anxiety symptoms, including being quick to anger, and having irritability, nervousness, or insomnia. In any case, if you present with these symptoms, I want you to get your hormones assessed by a physician, so you can see how balanced you are physically. This will also help to clarify whether your symptoms are caused exclusively by a hormonal imbalance, or if life stressors are causing some of your symptoms.

Achieving physical balance may help with emotional balance as well, because estrogen can increase serotonin. Serotonin is a brain chemical (a neurotransmitter) that is associated with good mood, happiness, and a general feeling of being upbeat and positive. If you've taken or heard of SSRIs (selective serotonin reuptake inhibitors), a popular type of antidepressant, you know those are the medications that are most often prescribed in an attempt to increase your serotonin levels. So, if you've got a doctor who's working on your hormones, and you're also working with a psychiatrist for the psychotropic medications, then you'll definitely want to make sure that their plans are coordinated. You might not need the same dose of your psychotropic medication if your hormones are balanced. Make sure that the doctor who prescribes your psychotropic medications is aware if you're taking birth control pills, as they can cause depression in some women.

Thyroid Hormones

If you've got PCOS, someone has probably tested your **Thyroid Hormones (T3 and T4, TSH)**. And while we generally don't like to tell our doctors what to do, in this case, if you haven't been tested, I suggest you ask to be tested. The thyroid gland is incredibly important. It's like a thermostat for your body, and it controls metabolic action throughout your entire body. So, if your thyroid is not functioning properly (either too high or too low), everything is affected, both physically and emotionally. Hypothyroidism (low thyroid) is particularly common in women with PCOS, and can be present at a sub-clinical level for a long time before you're actually diagnosed with a problem. You might notice symptoms like unrelenting fatigue, difficulty getting out of bed in the morning, weight gain, lack of energy during the day, lack of motivation, memory problems, and concentration problems. There are multiple causes of hypothyroidism, including auto-immune causes, so it's important to get tested and treated by someone who's knowledgeable, because the treatments can be quite nuanced. Usually, that's an endocrinologist. The most common fix for hypothyroidism is a tiny pill containing thyroid replacement that is taken daily for life. When dosed properly, you should experience no side effects at all – just a return to more normal functioning and maybe a little weight loss.

Cortisol is commonly called the stress hormone, and it's part of the adrenal system. You may have heard someone talk about "adrenal exhaustion," or been diagnosed with it yourself. Adrenal exhaustion is not a western medicine diagnosis, but it's a very common diagnosis in the alternative medicine world. What they're talking about is being under chronic stress and wearing out that gland. The result is anxiety, anger, irritability, depression, fatigue, forgetfulness, and a short temper. Basically, you lack the physical ability to counter the stress. This contributes to a further breakdown of the whole system and leads to – guess what? – more stress and more symptoms!

DHEA is a hormone secreted by the ovaries and adrenal system. It helps us maintain a positive mood and attitude, have good energy, keep up immunity, and have a healthy libido. It is a precursor to both testosterone and estrogen. Abnormally low levels of DHEA are implicated in depression. So if you're feeling depressed, anxious, tired, totally uninterested in sex, and you're catching colds or having the flu all the time, there's a good chance that your levels of DHEA are inadequate. In order to increase the DHEA in your body, you should be looking to diet and fish oil supplements. I encourage you to do some further research to assess the benefits for yourself. Because of the far-reaching effects of DHEA, I recommend supplementing directly with DHEA only under the direction of a health care professional.

Melatonin, Vitamin D, and Sleep

Melatonin helps with sleep cycles, jetlag, and time-zone adjustments. It also works in conjunction with Vitamin D, which is your morning wake-up call. People with seasonal affective disorder (SAD), or who don't have the disorder, but seem to be particularly affected by seasonally related changes (not enough sunlight), are likely experiencing a melatonin deficiency. Melatonin is involved in relaxing the muscles and nerves at night, and is also an anti-oxidant. Mood symptoms related to melatonin deficiency include night-time anxiety, nervousness, irritability, insomnia, and depression.

Many people try melatonin hoping for a quick fix for their insomnia, and for many people, it does work that way. For those of us who say "melatonin–hmph!"– you might want to try it again. I've found that, even where it doesn't appear to have an immediate benefit, it will often contribute to improved quality of sleep over time. There are people who will tell you that melatonin is to be used for a short-term fix only, and that it will damage the body's ability to produce its own. In the absence of definitive proof either way, I recommend intermittent use of melatonin only. Just know that if you've been taking it for a while, and stop using it, it may take time for your body to be able to gear up and start producing melatonin on its own again. Note also that melatonin production naturally declines over time, which explains why so many older people have sleep problems, or seem to need less sleep. Additionally, it seems that most melatonin self-prescribers are using too large a dose and at the wrong time. Half a milligram (500 mcg), taken a few hours before bedtime, is recommended if falling asleep is your problem. If waking during the night is a problem, then a second tiny dose (500 mcg again) right at bedtime may be helpful. A few weeks of melatonin usage may be enough to reset your internal time clock.

Vitamin D is not actually a vitamin, although it used to be classified as one. It is now classified as a hormone, which basically means something that affects your other cells. It's involved in bone health (in balance with calcium), cell generation/regeneration, insulin sensitivity and blood sugar regulation, and binds to over 200 genes throughout the body. Note, if you're wearing sunscreen, you're probably not getting enough Vitamin D. Your Vitamin D level can be easily tested by your doctor, and supplementation is easy, inexpensive, and effective. Getting your Vitamin D level into the healthy zone may help improve sleep and decrease depression.

Challenge #1: Assess Your Real Stress Levels

Most of us are dealing with greater stress levels than people could have imagined even 100 years ago. To assess the intensity of your personal stress level, look up the Holmes-Rahe Stress Inventory (https://www.stress.org/holmes-rahe-stress-inventory/) and check out your score. Note that even positive life events cause stress – and your body doesn't really know the difference! I think of this scale as a reality checking tool. Right now, just keep that in mind as you continue reading.

Journaling Prompt: Handwritten journals are preferred over online journals, because the brain/emotional connection is stronger. This exercise is a three-page dialogue between you and your stress. Don't worry if you feel stuck, or this feels silly at first. Start out easy and see how it evolves when you ask stress what sort of messages it has for you, how you can help it, or how it plans to help you. Here's an example of how I might start:

Gretchen: Hey, stress, how are you doing?

Stress: Are you kidding? I'm loving it. I'm totally in charge here.

Gretchen: Well, yeah, you're pretty powerful, but I'm sure I'm in charge here!

Stress: Oh no. Take a look at what's going on in your body...

CHAPTER 4
Food, Eating, and Eating Disorders

M any PCOS professionals have observed a very high prevalence of eating disordered behavior in women with PCOS; in my practice, I'd put it at close to 100%. It's understandable how eating disorders develop, arising out of the frustrating almost impossibility of losing weight, which leads to increasing exercise and decreasing food consumption/restricting in order to lose. Additionally, women who are under high levels of stress, living in trauma-filled homes, or who face shifting and punitive cultural ideals about desirable body size and physical appearance are more likely to develop an eating disorder. The most common forms of eating disorders in women with PCOS are Anorexia Nervosa, Bulimia Nervosa, Binge Eating Disorder, and Orthorexia.

Anorexia Nervosa

Anorexia is defined by an abnormally low body weight, an obsessive desire to lose weight, and a distorted body image. People with anorexia, who are mostly women, place a high value on controlling their body image and weight, often to the exclusion of other behaviors. They may use laxatives, vomiting, diuretics, enemas, food restriction, and/or excessive exercise to accomplish their goals. Side effects may include esophageal erosion, other gastrointestinal issues, loss of body hair or development of a fine, fuzzy down-like hair on the body, reduced muscle mass, cardiac damage, dental damage, and even death. According to the National Eating Disorders Association, 4% of people with Anorexia die as a direct result. In my experience, it is least likely that a PCOS patient with an eating disorder will have Anorexia, but it is certainly not impossible.

Bulimia Nervosa

Bulimia is potentially as deadly as Anorexia, but it is often treated as a less-serious eating disorder. Signs and symptoms may also include being preoccupied with your body shape and weight, being fearful of weight gain, feeling out of control around eating behavior, eating until the point of discomfort or pain, and eating an unusually large volume of food in one sitting. People with Bulimia are often of normal weight, but may also be overweight, despite using methods like vomiting, food avoidance, compensatory calorie restriction, or misusing laxatives or diuretics.

Binge Eating Disorder

This disorder (BED) is actually slightly deadlier than the others. Suicide is often a risk in patients with BED. In order to have an actual diagnosis, you must eat more food in a short period of time than most people would eat under similar circumstances, and feel out of control of the eating, like you can't stop or limit the amount. It also involves eating much more rapidly than normal, eating until you are uncomfortably full, eating when you're not hungry, eating when you're alone (out of embarrassment), and feeling disgusted, depressed, or guilty afterwards. The patient must also feel "marked distress" and the binging must occur at least once a week for three months. Unlike the other eating disorders, purging or other compensating behaviors are not part of BED.

Orthorexia Nervosa

There is another category of eating-disordered behavior that isn't officially an eating disorder. It's called Orthorexia, and it interests me because many women with PCOS fall into this category, and it evolves into a full-scale eating disorder, as described above. It's a problematic behavior that starts by choosing to eliminate some blatantly unhealthy foods or categories of foods – say, high-fructose corn syrup or refined sugar. We can all get behind that concept. Everyone knows those things are pretty bad, so there's a lot of support for it. The goal is usually defined as consuming a diet that includes only pure, healthy foods. Then, perhaps, there's the addition of other foods or categories of foods to the list – white bread, dairy, hydrogenated fats, or gluten. That's getting a little narrower, but many positive arguments can be made for the elimination of these things, and the goal is still a pursuit of healthy living, so again, there's lots of support for it. But what's insidious is that, like any other eating-disordered behavior, there's now an element of power that's derived from being able to limit one's diet. There's also a great deal of cultural reward and support for these behaviors, and innumerable products and plans to help support these choices, such as the explosion of gluten-free products in recent years.

Additionally, there may be benefits like weight loss or better digestive functioning that motivate someone to keep going. By the way, women with PCOS suffer from an inordinately high number of digestive disorders as well. The thought process is: "If I'm feeling so much better, maybe I'll feel EVEN better if I cut out _____, _____, or _____". Eventually, you may find yourself with a very strange and limited diet. I'm thinking of a client whose primary source of protein was watermelon. (Did you know there's 0.14 ounces of protein in a whole watermelon? Can you see how this might be a problem?) Many vegans and raw-food enthusiasts fit in this category, but non-vegetarians can fit in this category too. *Please note that I am not labeling veganism an eating disorder; if practiced with caution, it may be both healthy and suitable for an individual.* It's actually a form of Obsessive Compulsive Disorder, and is often accompanied by extreme anxiety. It can lead to malnourishment or the development of full-blown Anorexia. It's not healthy; it's just pretending to be healthy.

Treatment for Eating Disorders

Treatments for all eating disorders include psychotherapy, dietary management and retraining, and learning how to exercise in a healthy way. Stress management techniques and relationship skills are also part of a good eating disorder treatment plan. Perfectionistic tendencies, a strong need to be in control, and difficulty expressing needs and feelings may also be addressed. If you are abusing laxatives or diuretics or vomiting, you must stop. Sometimes inpatient treatment is necessary to achieve complete remission. Lifelong vigilance is required, since acute stress may reactivate old eating-disordered behaviors.

The work in psychotherapy includes addressing anxiety and compulsive behaviors, strengthening relationships, and working through repressed feelings of anger, worthlessness, and shame. Binging is typically a way to relieve tension or numb out from negative feelings, so learning how to cope with those "undesirable" feelings is part of the treatment. Many people with BED also experience isolation, depression, moodiness, and irritability. They may feel disgusted about their body size and have been teased about their bodies while they were growing up.

Women with PCOS have BED so often that it's one of my standard screening questions. The issues of body shaming and repeated attempts and failures to control cravings and consumption may lead to the self-imposition of increasingly rigid rules and boundaries around food, and eating behaviors that ultimately manifest into a full-blown eating disorder. And all this time spent managing, worrying about, preparing, researching, sourcing, hiding, and manipulating food takes up so much of your energy. I believe that without treating the eating disorder, it is impossible to effectively treat depression and anxiety, which is why it's so important to be candid about your eating behaviors and concerns with anyone who is treating you.

In the next chapter, we'll be looking at sleep related issues that frequently affect women with PCOS. I give a lot of attention to both food and sleep because they're our core self-care functions – without food and sleep, you're not going to get very far in life!

Challenge #2: Keep a Food/Mood Log for a Week

Food is powerful medicine, but it can also be just as bad as any drug. Developing a thorough understanding of how what you eat affects how you feel is important to your long-term success in managing PCOS. It doesn't matter what day of the week you start, but keep a food/mood journal for a full seven days on a normal week – not when you're vacationing, going to a conference, etc. Include the day, date, time, what you ate, how much you ate, and how you felt before and after you ate it. At the end of the week, see if you can discern any patterns, such as always eating when you're angry, not eating when you're sad, etc. There's a free download of a food/mood log available on PCOSwellness.com.

Journaling Prompt: Write two to three pages at the end of the week, after you've completed your food/mood log. Note any patterns you observed, how you felt about tracking (were you angry, ashamed, annoyed?) and what, if anything, you plan to change as a result of doing this exercise. There are no right or wrong answers – just observations.

CHAPTER 5
Insomnia and Other Sleep Disorders

There are only two things you should be doing in bed: sleeping and having sex. This chapter addresses the former. When you engage in other activities such as reading, playing games, watching TV, or eating, your brain learns to associate the bed and the bedroom with waking, alertness, and engagement, all of which are contrary to the goal of sleep. Multi-tasking, electric lights, electronic devices and non-stop schedules are all contributors to sleep issues. That takes a huge toll on sleep, and there's no escaping the fact that we really all do need approximately eight hours per night to ensure optimal functioning. In fact, two-thirds of people have occasional sleep issues, and one quarter have chronic sleep problems.

Current research, and my clinical experience, indicate that nine hours may be more suitable for women with PCOS than the commonly recommended seven or eight hours per night. Many women with PCOS, as with most things, experience sleep issues far more often than the average woman. Not only does this mean you won't be well-rested, energetic, and ready to get out there and exercise and engage in the world, it may lead to some more serious consequences.

The serious fallout of chronic sleep deprivation or disruption shows up in a variety of ways. Your immune system is negatively affected by lack of sleep, leaving you more vulnerable to infection and other stress-related illnesses. Poor sleep can cause or contribute to weight gain, which of course doesn't enhance anyone's health. It may be also be a symptom or cause of heart disease, particularly if you have undetected or untreated sleep apnea. Occasional insomnia is annoying, but it won't really harm you. Extended insomnia, however, can cause or contribute to depression. It can make people with anxiety disorders more anxious as well. You may literally be wearing out your body faster than you should be.

Types of Sleep Disorders

In addition to the best known sleep disorder, Insomnia (where you have difficulty falling asleep, staying asleep, or getting good quality sleep for more than a month), there are a number of other sleep disorders, including:

Hypersomnia – excessive sleepiness for at least a month. It often occurs in conjunction with Obstructive Sleep Apnea and/or obesity. Hypersomnia is a symptom of depression as well.

Nightmare disorder/night terrors – if you have recurrent nightmares or other frightening dreams that cause you to wake up feeling distressed or anxious, you may develop a cumulative fatigue that is actually a sleep disorder.

Breathing-related sleep disorders – you might have excessive daytime sleepiness or fatigue because of Obstructive Sleep Apnea. Symptoms include loud snoring, breathing pauses that disrupt sleep, sleep that doesn't refresh, and waking with a headache in the morning. There is a much higher occurrence of sleep apnea among women with PCOS, and sleep apnea can contribute to the development or exacerbation of heart disease and diabetes, among other issues. It's very important to see a pulmonologist or other sleep specialist for further assessment if you have these symptoms. Severe untreated sleep apnea may result in premature death.

Parasomnias/Sleepwalking – unusual movement-related behavior during sleep, often sleepwalking, getting up to eat while asleep (reported on some medications as well), or sometimes having sex during sleep without being aware of it. Restless leg syndrome, while not a psychological disorder, is a related medical disorder that can cause sleep disruption.

Dyssomnias – a broad term covering problems falling asleep, staying asleep, or sleeping too much – any time your amount, quality or sleep timing is off, it's called a dyssomnia. The more commonly used term Insomnia will tell any expert what they need to know though.

Narcolepsy is repeated irresistible attacks of refreshing sleep, along with some other symptoms. Although rare, it can be very dangerous (say, when driving, caring for a child, or in a pool, etc.), because of its surprise nature.

Circadian Rhythm Sleep Disorder – this form of insomnia most often occurs as a result of jet lag, shift work, or after having a significant disruption to your sleep schedule, like pulling an all-nighter before a big exam. Basically, your body is just so OFF, it can't or won't get to sleep.

Substance-induced sleep disorders – this results from the use, or recent discontinuation of substances, causing sleep disruptions (for example, if you've been relying on marijuana to help you sleep, stopping smoking it may result in Insomnia). Substances can include marijuana, alcohol, multiple prescription medications, and illicit drugs.

Sleep disorders related to a general medical condition – this occurs when your sleep disorder comes about as a result, or side effect, of a medical condition. Several chronic diseases disrupt sleep. These include kidney disease, diabetes and pre-diabetes (because of irregularities in blood sugars, as well as the frequent need to get up to urinate during the night), cardiovascular disease, thyroid disease, heartburn, gastrointestinal disorders like Crohn's disease, neurological diseases, and pain disorders. Many medications used to treat medical conditions may also disrupt sleep. Statins, beta-blockers, and SSRIs are common culprits in the prescription-related issues.

Getting Help for Your Sleep Problems

If you have any of these symptoms, behaviors, or concerns, it's important to get assessed by a professional, or a team of professionals. Your doctor could be the first stop and the person to refer you for an overnight sleep study at a sleep lab if Obstructive Sleep Apnea is suspected. Your therapist can also assess for sleep issues and provide behavioral treatments and lifestyle modifications, as well as make appropriate medical referrals. If you have complex or long-standing sleep issues, you might need to add a sleep specialist, typically a pulmonologist.

Surprising Negative Effects of Poor Sleep

To expand upon what I listed above, the effects of sleep problems are system-wide and often dire. It's not just about being tired.

Your immune system is negatively affected by lack of sleep. When you already have a chronic illness, such as PCOS and its many offshoots, you are more vulnerable to infectious diseases anyway. The body is chronically taxed and has fewer resources available to fight off other germs, bacteria, and viruses.

Poor sleep can cause or contribute to weight gain. This is related both to the effects of cortisol (your body is always in some sort of panic mode and sending out surges of cortisol) as well as being so tired from lack of sleep that you:

- Don't get up early enough to exercise.
- Can't last late enough in the day to do planned exercise.
- Don't exercise at all, regardless of time of day.
- Eat more, typically carbohydrates, in an effort to produce serotonin and get the energy that comes from a glucose surge to make yourself feel better.

If you're thinking: "wow, that sounds like a vicious circle," you are correct. Numerous studies have linked Insomnia, Obstructive Sleep Apnea and other sleep disorders with an increased risk of heart disease. Since PCOS already gives you an increased risk of heart disease, I say, why add fuel to the fire?

Insomnia is insidious in that it can cause or exacerbate depression. Chronic Insomnia can actually cause a full-blown major depressive episode, which is much harder to treat than a mild depressive episode. It also takes longer. If you're already dealing with depression, it can make it worse, or make it harder to get rid of. If you have bipolar disorder, insomnia can be extra dangerous, as it can trigger manic or hypomanic episodes.

Insomnia can make you really grumpy, which has negative effects on your relationships, your work life, and your family life. When you're irritable, people don't like to be around you, and you don't like to be around them. This may lead to isolation which is yet another symptom of depression.

Are you now convinced that you've **got** to do something about your sleep? *Chapter 17: Improving Sleep* is about how to address sleep problems on your own. I'm convinced that when you see how easily you can improve your sleep, and how much better you feel when your sleep is improved, you will want to keep up with these changes. This includes information about what you're consuming and correcting or enhancing the sleep environment. There's also some really interesting information about what you eat and drink, when you consume it, and how it affects your sleep. There are some surprising consequences of sugar, caffeine, dairy, and alcohol. The great news is, these are all things you can experiment with on your own. You don't need a doctor to tell you to drink less coffee and see if it helps you sleep – but I'm going to do that anyway!

Challenge #3: Sleep More

This one should sound good to almost everyone. Your assignment is to get 30 minutes more sleep every night. I told you it was easy! Take note of how you feel.

Bonus points: At least once this week, get 60 minutes of extra sleep, preferably by going to bed earlier, not sleeping in later. Take note of how you feel.

Journaling Prompt: Make a list of all the things that interfere with your getting a consistent good night's sleep. Brainstorm some ways that you can begin changing the biggest problems.

CHAPTER 6
Mood Disorders

This is a bit of an over-simplification, but mood disorders are mostly different combinations and degrees of depression and anxiety or mania – unhealthy highs or lows in other words. This negatively affects quality of life, contributes to poor health outcomes, and may even be fatal. This chapter addresses depression, anxiety, and bipolar disorder. Psychosis, which affects far fewer people, is not addressed here due to space limitations.

Depression

We've all seen the advertisements on television, showing images of lethargic, sad-eyed men and women, dragging themselves around slowly. The background is gray and mournful music is playing. It feels like a funeral. While this is an artistic or symbolic representation of depression, it's also a pretty accurate representation of the feeling of depression.

Depression is a significant health problem. According to the World Health Organization, depression affects 350 million people worldwide. In America, almost 7% of the population has depression. More than 60% of women with PCOS have depression, dysthymia, or other mood disorders. It's normal to be sad occasionally, but it's definitely not normal to be depressed.

Furthermore, depression isn't something that just affects your mood. There are physical and behavioral impacts and consequences of untreated depression, including increased pain, reduced pain tolerance, inadequate self-care, engaging in attempts to self-medicate (with drugs, alcohol, or food), headaches, muscular aches, gastrointestinal distress, increased clumsiness and accidents, poor surgical outcomes, increased risk of premature death, and of course, suicide. For all those reasons, it's important to get treatment for your depression.

Depression, or Major Depressive Disorder, is diagnosed when you have the majority of these symptoms:

- Depressed mood most of the day, nearly every day, for at least two weeks. In children and adolescents (and often, in men), an irritable mood is the main symptom. Due to higher androgen levels, irritability may be a prominent feature of depression in women with PCOS too.
- Dramatically diminished interest or pleasure in all or most activities, most of the day, nearly every day.
- Significant weight loss or gain (more than five pounds in a month) when not dieting, or noteworthy decrease or increase in appetite nearly every day.
- Insomnia (not sleeping) or Hypersomnia (sleeping far too much, well over the average of eight hours/day) nearly every day.
- Psychomotor agitation or retardation nearly every day, meaning that you look agitated to other people, or notably slowed down.
- Fatigue or loss of energy nearly every day.
- Feelings of worthlessness, or excessive or inappropriate guilt nearly every day.
- Diminished ability to think or concentrate, or indecisiveness, nearly every day.
- Recurrent thoughts of death (not just fear of dying), including recurrent thoughts of suicide without a specific plan, a suicide attempt, or a specific plan for committing suicide.

Dysthymia

Dysthymia is sometimes mistakenly described as "depression light," but it is far from benign. It can have similarly devastating effects on your quality of life. Dysthymia is similar to Major Depressive Disorder but is less severe and may be more chronic in nature. You'll note that most of the symptom list is the same; however, you need to have fewer symptoms to qualify for the diagnosis:

- Depressed mood most of the day, for more days than not, as indicated either by your own reports, or the reports of others, for at least two years. Irritable mood may be a factor.
- Presence, while depressed, of two (or more) of the following:

    1. Poor appetite or overeating
    2. Insomnia or Hypersomnia
    3. Low energy or fatigue
    4. Low self-esteem
    5. Poor concentration or difficulty making decisions
    6. Feelings of hopelessness

One of the most important differences is the presence of low self-esteem, which is quite common among women with PCOS.

Likelihood of Developing Depression or Dysthymia

If you've had Depression once, there's a much greater likelihood that you'll have it again during your lifetime. And, people with Dysthymia are also at much greater risk for developing Depression later in life. Those numbers look something like this:

- Single depressive episode: 50% chance of recurrence.
- Two episodes: 70% chance of recurrence.
- Three episodes: 90% chance of recurrence.

Having a family history of depression increases your risk for developing Depression. The risk is more meaningful if the family member is a parent or sibling, but still meaningful if someone in your extended family has depression. This is also true of Bipolar Disorder, Schizophrenia and anxiety disorders. It may not have been called Depression, but if someone in your family suffered from "the blues" or "melancholia," died by suicide, had bipolar disorder or was manic depressive, or was generally remembered as reclusive, sad, and withdrawn, there's a good chance that you've got Depression in your family. However, just because you're part of that gene pool, it doesn't mean you're guaranteed to develop the same diseases or conditions.

"Double Depression" and Other Forms of Depression

To further complicate matters, you can also suffer from a variety of forms, sub-types, and variations of Depression, including:

Double Depression – which is when you have both Major Depression and Dysthymia at the same time. This is chronic, low-level depression topped off with a more severe episode of Depression. It is not a formal diagnosis, but I find it extremely helpful in understanding depression.

Atypical Depression – women with PCOS who have Atypical Depression might actually feel better temporarily when something good happens, but then go back to feeling depressed quickly. It's probably under-diagnosed, but Atypical Depression may be the most common form of depression.

Adjustment disorder with depressed mood – when a major life event requires a lot of changes that produce stress, it may temporarily give you symptoms of depression.

Postpartum depression – approximately 10% of mothers may have depression after giving birth (there is a milder form referred to as "postpartum blues" and a much more severe form, "postpartum psychosis"). A history of Dysthymia or Depression in yourself or other relatives may increase the chances of developing postpartum depression.

Premenstrual dysphoric disorder - this occurs when a woman has depressive symptoms one week prior to menstruation that disappear following menstruation. Charting symptoms is an easy way to help diagnosis this one. Using prescription medication for part of the month may help.

Seasonal affective disorder – this is a pattern of depression related to the seasons and a lack of sunlight. It occurs during the fall and winter seasons and disappears during the spring and summer seasons. It is more common in areas that experience extended periods of gloomy weather (which decreases sunlight), or where there are extreme seasonal disruptions in the day/night rhythms, such as in the Netherlands. Use of a light box for a few months per year may help alleviate symptoms.

Bipolar disorder (formerly known as manic-depressive disorder) – is characterized by mood swings ranging from depression to mania or hypomania. The depressive symptoms often include feeling suicidal. The manic or hypomanic symptoms can include other extreme, impulsive, and unsafe behaviors. Medication is almost always required to effectively manage bipolar disorder.

Bereavement (grief) is perfectly normal, and is not depression, but is sometimes misdiagnosed as depression, or can become depression if it doesn't resolve fairly quickly.

Anxiety

Women with PCOS also report significantly higher levels of anxiety. Anxiety is excessive worry about normal life situations. It may be a worry about your capabilities, health, appearance, or ability to perform well. You can also have physical symptoms such as sweating, nausea, or diarrhea.

For a diagnosis of Generalized Anxiety Disorder, you would need to have worry that is hard to control and affects your regular daily activities, causing problems at work, school or in relationships. You would also have at least three of the following symptoms: feeling edgy or restless; tiring easily or feeling more fatigued than usual; feeling like your mind goes blank or you have difficulty concentrating; irritability; frequent muscle aches and soreness or difficulty sleeping.

It's also important to note that sometimes medical conditions can cause anxiety symptoms. Substances such as prescription medication, alcohol, or recreational drugs can also cause anxiety symptoms. Other mental disorders may include anxiety as part of the symptoms. It's important to consult with a skilled health psychologist when trying to determine the cause(s) of your anxiety.

What if You Only Have Some of the Symptoms?

If you've read through the symptom lists and are thinking "a lot of this sounds like me, but not all of it, so I'm not really sure if I have a problem or not," you may benefit from further assessment, exploration, and working with a therapist because I've only listed the most common forms of depression and anxiety here. There are many variations on these disorders, and there's even a whole separate category for when:

- You have some symptoms, but not enough to qualify for the diagnosis (yet).
- It's unclear when your depression or anxiety started, or how long you've had it.
- It's clear you have a mood disorder, but we don't know if this is the first, second, or 20ᵗʰ time.
- Some of your symptoms fit in one diagnostic category and some of them fit in at least one other category, so we can't assign a diagnosis.

The bottom line is this – if you're suffering from several of these symptoms or feelings, you may well have some form of mood disorder. It's important to talk to a skilled mental health professional who can assess your symptoms and life circumstances to see if you have a mood disorder, how bad it is, and what to do about it.

Preventing Mood Disorders

If you don't already have a mood disorder, that's great - let's try to keep it that way. Here are some things you can do that are preventative:

- Get regular mental health screenings at least once a year. Just like going to the dentist to get your teeth cleaned helps prevent tooth and gum decay, your brain can use a little preventative maintenance. Mood disorders are much easier to treat and resolve when they're caught early on.
- Maintain a positive outlook. Surround yourself with people who are generally happy, optimistic, and think about the future in a positive way. Keep a gratitude list. Stop talking about things in negative terms. Studies show that the more we focus on the positive and on feeling grateful, the less likely we are to develop symptoms of mental health problems.
- Be honest with your doctors, friends, and family if you are having any signs or symptoms of Depression, especially if you're feeling suicidal. Suicide is highly preventable, especially when the symptoms are caught and treated quickly.
- Engage in healthy self-care practices that promote feeling good in your mind and body. This book is full of suggestions.
- Avoid the things that make you feel bad. Be especially vigilant about alcohol consumption, because alcohol is a depressant. If you're already feeling depressed, adding alcohol will NOT help, and it puts you at higher risk for suicide as well. Avoid negative people, stressful environments, and even the news.

Wishing Isn't Enough to Make It Go Away

You might feel like you're being a whiner if you complain about these symptoms to your doctor or someone else. I disagree. I would much rather have you tell me about your symptoms early on than wait until you're so depressed or anxious you can't leave the house or are thinking about killing yourself. Your doctors want to help. We all need to know what's going on with you, or we can't do anything to help improve things for you. Being proactive in letting an expert know that something feels really wrong is good self-care.

If you're worried that mood disorders are over-diagnosed, and you're just going to get handed a prescription, sure, there's a possibility of that. But again, it's better to be safe when it comes to Depression and other Mood Disorders. My guess is that Depression is under-diagnosed, because depressed people often keep to themselves. Isolation is a symptom of Depression. Depressed and anxious people often skip going go to the doctor regularly, or don't follow-through on treatments. That being said, I do think anti-depressants are over-prescribed.

I also think that the terms "depression," "trauma," "psychotic," and "bipolar" are overused, often inappropriately. All those words have specific clinical meanings, so I'm going to ask a lot of questions if you walk into my office saying: "I'm feeling totally psychotic today." The words have become integrated into our culture, our collective references, and, in the process, have lost meaning. We forget that it's quite normal to feel bad, sad, angry, or out of sorts. Life is uneven.

Challenge #4: Make a Symptom List

After reading this chapter, compile a list of the mood symptoms you've identified as good descriptions of how you feel. Make an appointment to see your doctor or therapist (or find one if you don't already have one), so that you can discuss your symptoms and the best way to get help with them.

Journaling prompt: Take a few minutes to respond to the question "What do you think your life would be like if you didn't have anxiety or depression?" Remember that this journal is only for you. Use this time to start envisioning a healthier, happier life, where PCOS-related mood disorders aren't ruling your life.

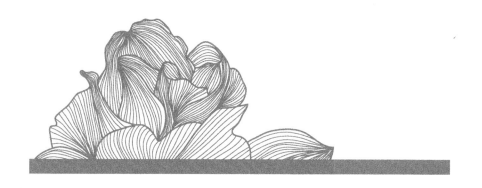

Part Two:

How to Live Better with PCOS

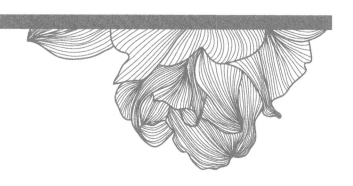

CHAPTER 7
Integrative Model

I have often said that I am a bad scientist because I don't always apply a treatment, wait a few weeks or months for results, and then adjust and start over with the waiting and assessment period. What I've learned over the years is that women come to see me when they are feeling miserable, overwhelmed, unheard, frustrated, and depressed about dealing with their PCOS. The phrase I often hear is "I'm sick and tired of being sick and tired." They want, need, and deserve to get better quickly.

I believe that an integrative approach to healthcare management is the only thing that works for women with PCOS, because our problems occur in all systems of the body and changes in one area will affect other areas. It is not uncommon for women with PCOS to have chronic pain issues, digestion and bowel issues, eating disorders, insomnia, allergies, and a host of other symptoms that affect more than one part or system in the body. An integrative approach is one that treats the whole woman, not just her ovaries, her hair growth, or her eating behaviors. I take a multi-pronged approach right from the start, with the philosophy being "let's do what it takes, as fast as possible, to get you feeling better."

I start by assessing medical issues, life stress, sleep, nutrition, exercise, and other psychological issues. While I begin psychotherapy immediately, medical issues must also be treated as a priority. Without understanding the baseline metabolic issues presenting in your particular version of PCOS, and starting to make the appropriate medical adjustments, it will slow down treatment for mood disorders. I understand that many women have had bad experiences with doctors. Many women have told me about fat-shaming (which hurts even worse if you know you've been diligent about diet and exercise), fear-inducing warnings, and doctors who are dismissive of their symptoms, or refuse to consider any treatment approach except medication. If you don't have a good endocrinologist, I'll make a referral to someone local who understands PCOS emotionally as well as physically, or teach you how to find a suitable physician.

I typically coordinate care with a woman's doctors, nutritionist, and other medical professionals and caregivers such as acupuncturists, and even knowledgeable personal trainers. I talk to each of those professionals about my approach to PCOS management, their approach, what our respective roles are, and how best we can support each other in caring for our mutual patient.

It's important to find a medical provider you're comfortable with, because PCOS care is more of a marathon than a sprint. This is definitely not a "once and done" problem. I believe that not only will you be a more compliant (and thus healthier) patient when you like your doctor, some psychological distress will be relieved when you truly like your doctor and feel liked and respected by your doctor in return. Also, everyone who is taking care of you needs to be aware of your goals as the patient, which may be very different from what we think your goals should be. For example, your goal might be "weight loss no matter how it has to happen," while your dietician's goal is "health at any size." If we're working toward different outcomes, your treatment is going to be inconsistent and perhaps frustrating.

In addition to an endocrinologist, I may make other referrals to people that I think will be necessary or helpful, and I always check this with you first to see if you're ready for some more change. Sometimes, one big change is all a woman can really handle at that moment, and that's okay. It can be grueling to make appointments, fill out forms, deal with insurance, take time off from work, and tell your whole story again to someone new. I keep the whole long-term picture in mind and discuss priorities with you so that we start acting as a team right from the beginning of treatment.

Because I feel so strongly about having a whole team of helpers on the PCOS journey, I want to make sure that we're talking about medical issues regularly during therapy. I need to know about medication changes or major dietary or exercise changes, for example, because those things can have a significant effect on your mood. I also provide a lot of education about why it's so important to have more than one doctor working on your health issues.

Hopefully, the idea of having a whole team contributing to your care makes sense. In the next chapter, I'll talk about how to assemble your optimal group of personal PCOS experts.

CHAPTER 8
Assembling Your Health Care Team

You may feel like you've already seen all the doctors you ever wanted to see, or maybe you haven't really started seeking care yet. Maybe you've just got the one doctor you've been seeing most of your life, who finally diagnosed you with PCOS. In any case, I recommend taking a strategic approach to assembling a health care team to help you cope with your PCOS. This may include medical doctors, alternative practitioners, and mental health practitioners. Ideally, you'll have a traditional western medical doctor and a naturopath or other complementary/alternative medicine practitioner to provide a possibly different perspective. Typical Western-style allopathic practitioners will take a specialized approach rather than an integrative approach to the body and mind. Naturopaths, chiropractors, holistic and integrative physicians, osteopaths, and similar providers tend to look at the body as a whole, incorporating much more information about diet, exercise, environment, life stressors, etc., which I think is really helpful. I believe in taking advantage of the best of both worlds.

Discuss it With an Expert

One of the most frequent and important pieces of advice I give is "discuss it with another expert." It's really valuable to have more than one opinion, especially with something as complicated as PCOS. There are many types of experts, and those who claim to be experts. Be mindful of who your experts are. A "nutritionist" who prescribes a weight loss diet of 300 calories a day may get results, may be popular with celebrities, and may also be entirely unreliable as an expert. I've seen a number of books about health and nutrition written by laypeople who found a way to lose weight that worked for them, or get over anxiety or ADHD. They slapped a clever name on it, marketed it like crazy, and made a bunch of money and gained some celebrity along the way. They may be experts on their own condition, but that doesn't make them experts for the rest of us.

Conversely, just because somebody's got a Ph.D. or M.D. after their name doesn't mean they're ideal experts either. We take nutrition advice from doctors who receive, on average, THIRTY minutes of nutritional training during their time in medical school. I'm thinking that's not such a good idea. We take spiritual advice from yoga teachers who have nothing more than a certificate program in yoga. I am not diminishing those who have legitimately developed large bodies of knowledge through independent study, but I urge you to consider the sources of your information carefully. Just because something's popular doesn't mean it's good and this applies to health advice probably more than any other advice, because the consequences of following bad information can be so dire.

This list is not meant to be exhaustive, as there are many specialists you may encounter along your health journey, but it includes the ones you're most likely to need for PCOS: an endocrinologist, gynecologist, internist or general practitioner, psychotherapist and dietician/nutritionist. I'll describe each of them below, along with why I think they're important, and some tips for making your selections.

Before You See the Doctor

Don't overwhelm yourself by going to several new doctors simultaneously. I can't emphasize this enough. It's like what happens when you go from zero to 60 on an exercise program, you get injured, and drop out. Start with the most basic, consult with them about necessary additions to your team and ask them to help you prioritize your needs. They will all want blood tests, medical history, and a personal examination, which can get exhausting. They will also make recommendations that may be in contradiction, and if you're not used to being a proactive medical consumer, it can easily become overwhelming.

For example, if your doctor thinks you have diabetes, that requires immediate attention. If your doctor thinks it's a good idea for you to go for a screening exam, like a mammogram, that you've been skipping for a while anyway, ask if it can wait a couple of months. The experience of revealing your entire medical history, as well as your often-naked body, to a bevy of new people is one best handled in bits and pieces. You may think you can handle it, but it's my personal experience and professional observation that adding too many doctors to your life all at once leads to feelings of frustration, fear, anxiety, and being overwhelmed. The net result may be shutting down, acting out, or giving up, all of which are counter-productive to your goal of getting better.

Although many doctors will be very persuasive about the urgency of their recommendations, you also have to take into consideration your lifestyle, insurance, finances, and personal preferences. If you're getting ready to head off for a month in Europe, this is not the time to try a new medication or, frankly, a new diet. This approach is long-term, and you will have the highest chances of success if you start when you're motivated and have a little time to dedicate to getting used to new behaviors, medications, or dietary changes.

If going to the doctor frightens or intimidates you in any way, take someone with you – someone you trust, who is comfortable in medical settings, and who can take some notes for you while you're talking to the doctor. Maybe even someone who can speak up on your behalf if it seems like your needs aren't being met, or you are becoming emotional. It doesn't have to be a person with medical training, but definitely find someone who doesn't freak out at the sight of blood (or old people, or lab coats, or whatever excuse people come up with).

You may also find it helpful to prepare a list of questions, in writing, in advance of the meeting with your doctor. This will help you and your doctor prioritize how your appointment time is spent and ensure that your most pressing concerns are addressed. You can write notes on the list, next to your questions, and go back to them for reference later.

When scheduling the first appointment with a new doctor, be sure to point out to the scheduler that you are a new patient if he or she doesn't ask, and mention that you have a number of concerns to address, so that adequate time is scheduled for your appointment. Initial appointments or "intakes" are usually about twice as long as standard follow-up appointments in a medical setting.

Ask if there are any records you should have sent over ahead of time, or that you can bring with you. Also ask if the doctor will require any blood work or urine at the time of the examination (there's nothing like having emptied your bladder right before an appointment and then being told you have to give a urine sample – pretty frustrating, and it even requires some patients to return to the office later).

Inquire about anything related to fees and insurance at this time, so that you're not caught by surprise when you get to the doctor's office. Ask how long the appointment is likely to take, if you need to arrive early to do paperwork or if paperwork can be faxed or mailed to you ahead of time, if there's an online patient portal you'll need to access, and about the parking situation. You can't control every detail, but if you know about the small stuff ahead of time, it makes the big stuff (actually talking to the doctor) much less intimidating.

Similarly, allow enough time for your appointment – plenty of time to get there, especially the first visit to a new doctor or medical building, some extra time in case the doctor is running late or you get sent to a nearby site for a blood draw, and time to process the experience afterwards. I don't mean you need an extra hour to sit in your car and de-stress, but give yourself some time over the next day or two to think about how the experience of meeting with this doctor felt overall, if the fit feels right, and if the doctor's recommendations feel manageable. The best doctor in town may not be the right fit for you if she only sees patients three days a week, starting at 10:00 a.m., and you have to be at work at 8:00 a.m., five days a week, to open your office.

Remember that modern medical offices are typically trying to be as efficient as possible, so they're working you into their structure, and not the other way around. This may not feel comfortable to you and, again, may not always be the best choice, even if the doctor has a stellar reputation. I'd rather have a tiny bit of inefficiency, and a whole lot more of the doctor's time and concern. The goal here is to find the right fit for you – a doctor you can have a long-term relationship with, who feels relatively comfortable to you emotionally, has a good technical skill set, and who genuinely has an interest in helping you with your PCOS.

If you've been avoiding doctors for a while, or had some bad experiences, you do have rights. Here's what should never happen with your doctor's appointment:

- The doctor forgets your appointment and/or just doesn't show up. Unless he or she is dead or seriously injured in an accident, your doctor should be there for scheduled appointments. The doctor's office should always have all your phone numbers, so they can contact you if the doctor is sick or otherwise unavailable.
- The doctor is running more than an hour late, and you don't receive a call from staff offering to reschedule you.
- The doctor touches parts of you that have nothing to do with why you're there (the ankle doctor wants to do a breast exam, for example). If you feel uncomfortable, ask why that part of the exam is necessary. If you're not comfortable with the answer, you have the right to refuse. It is normal, necessary, and appropriate for gynecologists, general practitioners, internists, and reproductive endocrinologists to do a complete gynecological exam and breast exam.
- The doctor yells at you, hits you, threatens you, shames you, or belittles you. I don't care if you've gained weight instead of lost it, failed to keep requested records, or taken your medication all wrong, it is never okay for a doctor to be physically or verbally abusive towards you. Doctors are or should be trained to approach patient "failures" with concern and persuasiveness. If the art of healthy communication seems lost on your doctor, find a new one. Like any other relationship, regardless of the person's level of education, or power differential, you deserve to be treated

with respect and compassion. A doctor who fails to treat you appropriately should be fired from your team and, if necessary, reported to the appropriate professional licensing board.

The Five Most Important Members of Your Medical Team

Your medical VIP list may differ from mine because of the specifics of your goals or condition, but usually I like to start with the basics and work into more specialized providers. For those of us with PCOS, that means an endocrinologist, a gynecologist, an internist or general practitioner, a psychotherapist, and a dietician. My rationale for each of these providers is explained below.

Endocrinologist – An endocrinologist is a doctor who specializes in the endocrine system, which has to do with your hormones. Balancing your hormones is the endocrinologist's goal. They typically address such diseases and concerns as diabetes, PCOS, and thyroid disorders. If you're like me and you've got all three, the endocrinologist is a great one-stop shop for most of your basic medical needs. Your endocrinologist will likely want you to have blood work on a quarterly basis and see you every few months to review your labs, discuss medications and strategies for symptom control, and coordinate your care with other specialists. If you have diabetes, your endocrinologist will manage your diabetes, and will often refer you to a dietician.

Not every endocrinologist is an expert in PCOS, or even particularly sensitive to the needs of PCOS patients. It's important to ask if PCOS patients constitute a large portion of the doctor's practice when you're doing your research. It's also important to know that this is a very numbers-oriented specialty, so lab tests will definitely be a frequent part of life, but it's also important to find a doctor who looks at your health from the perspective of the whole patient, not just your lab reports.

Gynecologist – A gynecologist treats the overall health of female patients, including problems and diseases of the female reproductive system. This includes breast and hormonal problems, urinary tract and pelvic disorders, and cancers affecting the reproductive system.

Gynecologists are also trained in obstetrics (delivering babies), although some choose not to practice obstetrics. For many otherwise healthy young women, the gynecologist serves as their primary care provider, although the gynecologist is actually a specialist.

The gynecologist is often the first to diagnose PCOS, and the first to prescribe treatment in the form of birth control pills. Because this is a doctor who's likely to prescribe powerful hormones to help regulate your system, you want to be sure that you can comfortably discuss the details of your health and sexual and reproductive concerns your gynecologist. Your gynecologist should be non-judgmental about your body, and gentle – after all, he or she is touching and looking at your most intimate parts.

The gynecologist will coordinate with the endocrinologist to make sure that they're taking a comprehensive, focused approach to medications and symptom management. Some gynecologists also provide assisted reproduction services. Many deliver babies, but many do not – if it's important to you to limit the number of doctors you see, and you're planning to have a baby, you may want to have a gynecologist who does currently practice obstetrics. It's also important to note that gynecology is actually a surgical specialty, whereas endocrinology is not – thus, the importance of having the two work with you simultaneously. If you need surgery for cyst removal, endometriosis, or related procedures, your gynecologist will most likely be the surgeon.

Internist or General Practitioner (GP) – An internist is an internal medicine doctor for adults, in the same way that pediatricians are general practitioners for children. A GP is a family doctor who treats a wide variety of conditions and patients. Both types of doctors are trained in general medicine practice, with working knowledge of all aspects of medicine. This doctor is the overall coordinator of your care and should be copied on all lab work. You will typically see this doctor for all concerns other than gynecology. Many internists and GPs manage PCOS, hypothyroidism, and straightforward cases of diabetes, but I strongly recommend having an endocrinologist for these issues. PCOS is too complex to be left to a doctor who doesn't have a deep understanding of the condition.

Internists and GPs often are also the first line of defense in detecting depression or other mental health issues, and may often prescribe anti-depressants. However, I recommend having a mental health professional coordinate your mental health care; your internist or GP simply doesn't have the time or training to address mental health concerns adequately. You should see your internist or GP once a year for a physical and to update medication records, and at any time when you're simply not feeling well, and not quite sure why. They will do preliminary lab work, diagnosis, and treatment, and make referrals to specialists if needed.

Psychotherapist – A psychotherapist, or therapist, is the mental health component of your health team. Because of the high rates of depression, anxiety, and other mood and eating disorders among women with PCOS, I think it's important for all of us to have a therapist.

Psychotherapists have many different professional designations – MFT, LCSW, Psychologist, Psychiatrist (addressed separately below) and in some states, LPC or a similar designation. All these professionals can be helpful in assessing mental health concerns, devising a treatment plan, and providing talk therapy, but there are differences in education and training. MFTs are Marriage and Family Therapists; they have a minimum of a master's degree and are often trained extensively in family systems approaches to mental health. LCSWs are Licensed Clinical Social Workers. They too have a minimum of a master's degree and have training that comprehensively addresses psycho-social needs such as the impact of housing, finances, access to medical care, etc. on one's well-being. Psychologists have a doctorate (either Ph.D. or Psy.D.) and may provide psychological testing in addition to psychotherapy. Psychiatrists have a medical degree (M.D.) and specialized training in psychiatry. Most therapists undergo a minimum of 3,000 hours of supervised practical training and pass national and local licensing exams. You can easily check online with most state's licensing boards to verify that your therapist is licensed and does not have a history of disciplinary action.

Nutritionist/Dietician – These terms are used interchangeably to describe someone who helps create nutritionally balanced eating plans, often for special populations, such as the elderly, pregnant women, people undergoing chemotherapy, etc. It's important for women with PCOS to work with someone skilled in PCOS dietetics, at least in the beginning, when trying to get pregnant, or when focusing on weight loss. If you can't find someone with PCOS-specific training, look for someone who works extensively with diabetes and pre-diabetes, as the guidelines are similar.

A registered dietician will have the designation R.D. after their name. Some nutritionists are also Certified Diabetes Educators (CDE), which means they have extra knowledge and training about insulin resistance. While all nutritionists offer advice about exercise as a part of weight management, some have additional training as Exercise Physiologists. Registered dieticians are trained to recognize eating disorders, signs of depression and suicidality, and other health issues.

Many people call themselves "nutritional counselors" or "health coaches" and there are numerous certificate programs that do not require the rigorous education and training that registered dieticians have. A nutritional counselor may not be able to provide you with appropriate care if you have a serious eating disorder or other complicated health issue. However, there are also many well-educated nutritional counselors and coaches who have specialized insight into PCOS and can be relied upon to provide quality information. Some of my favorites are listed in the Resources section in the back of this book.

Common Questions About Working with a Therapist

What is health psychology? Health psychologists are specialized psychologists (therapists) who not only have a doctorate in psychology, but also have specialized training and experience in medical issues, coping with chronic illness, making decisions about health care, and managing your relationships with your medical providers. They also help you deal with stress, grief, and loss.

There are so many different kinds of therapists out there - what's the best way to get therapy? Depending upon your budget, schedule, specialized needs, and/or insurance coverage, you may obtain therapy in a private outpatient setting, through a private or non-profit clinic, or from a community mental health clinic.

If I need a psychiatrist, how do I get a good one? The best way to find a good psychiatrist is through a therapist who understands your needs, personality, style, and can make an appropriate referral. The next best choice is through your primary health care provider, whether that's an MD or a naturopath or other alternative practitioner you trust. Insurance referral lists are usually the least useful way to obtain a good referral.

Does going to therapy mean I'm mentally ill? I believe it means you're mentally well, because you value yourself and your well-being enough to seek help when you need it. Even if you have a formal diagnosis, such as Depression, you are more than a set of symptoms. I see you as a person whose coping skills and inner resources can be enhanced, not as a disease.

Why would you want to talk to my doctor? Generally, your doctor addresses the needs of your body, and a therapist addresses the needs of your mind/soul/heart. But many psychological conditions are triggered by, worsened by, or mimic medical conditions. For example, Hypothyroidism (underactive thyroid) often produces symptoms that look like Depression – but can be easily corrected by taking a small dose of thyroid medication. As part of your mental health care, I might ask you to get a check-up or ask your doctor for some specific blood work so we can ensure proper treatment of your entire mind/body.

Other Physicians and Licensed Professionals

In addition to the above medical, psychological, and nutritional professionals, there are other doctors you will likely use at some point in your PCOS journey.

The **Dermatologist** is your skin-care expert. In addition to providing an annual full-body check for skin cancers, and anti-aging treatments, your dermatologist treats diseases of the skin, including conditions related to the hair, such as excess facial hair and hair loss on the head. If you're always itchy or rashy, see a dermatologist. Yeast overgrowth is a common cause of rashes, and extra likely to occur if you have folds of excess skin or fat, or if you are diabetic.

Dermatologists can assist with PCOS-related acne, acanthosis nigricans (the dark skin in the soft folds of the neck, underarms, etc.), hirsutism (excess hair on your face, chin, nipples, abdomen, etc.), hair loss (male pattern balding), removal of skin tags, and other skin conditions. At minimum, see the dermatologist once a year for a full-body skin cancer check. An easy guideline to remember is that you should get your "birthday suit" checked on your birthday.

Cardiologists treat your heart and circulatory system. It has become "best practice" for diabetics of any age to be screened by a cardiologist. In my opinion, PCOS, with its similar insulin resistance, should also generate an automatic referral to a cardiologist for evaluation, but your doctor may have a different opinion or standard of care. Heart disease and cholesterol problems are more common among PCOS patients, develop earlier, and develop with more severity than for the general population. In particular, if you have a family history of heart disease, it is important to add a cardiologist to your health care team early on because a great deal of damage can be prevented with proper care. Initial screenings include a health history, review of health habits related to your heart, like exercise, a physical examination, and recommendations to improve or protect your cardiovascular health.

Reproductive Endocrinologists (REs) are physicians who have specialized training in both gynecology and endocrinology. They not only handle infertility, often with the use of assisted reproductive technology, but they also handle complex endocrine imbalances that affect the reproductive system, such as PCOS. Typically, you will be referred to a RE if you're having trouble getting pregnant, staying pregnant, or having PCOS symptoms that are outside your gynecologist's skill set. The American Society of Reproductive Medicine (www.asrm.org) is a great place to start looking for a RE. Other resources include RESOLVE: The National Infertility Organization, www.resolve.org. Some REs are also board certified gynecologists and may be able to streamline some of your health care if you need procedures like cyst removal.

Psychiatrists are medical doctors who also have training in psychotropic medication and psychotherapy. They are generally oriented around the "chemical imbalance" theory of mental disorders and see their role as being prescription medication management. However, some of them do practice talk therapy. When necessary, I refer to psychiatrists, because I personally subscribe to a mixed theory about treatment effectiveness. I believe that sometimes the problem is caused by brain chemistry or hormonal imbalance, and sometimes it has more to do with life circumstances, stress, or coping styles.

Psychiatrists provide assessment, diagnosis, and treatment in the same ways that therapists do, but they are also licensed to prescribe medications (psychotropic medications are the set of drugs used to treat psychological disorders). Although any physician can dispense psychotropic medications, I always refer my clients to a psychiatrist for medication evaluations and medication management. Optimally, your psychiatrist will speak regularly with your psychotherapist to monitor your symptoms and ensure optimal improvement. Because many psychotropic medications may cause or contribute to weight gain and/ or insulin resistance, it's important to work with someone who is well-versed in all of the potential side effects of a medication and can discuss them with you realistically.

Psychotropic medications can also be dispensed by psychiatric nurse practitioners who often practice independently, but who work in conjunction with a psychiatrist. In addition to their nursing backgrounds, they have engaged in additional studies about medication and mental health issues. Their services may be substantially less expensive (typically less than half the price) than those of a psychiatrist. If money and/or lack of insurance is a significant issue, this is a valuable option. Also, depending upon your schedule and needs, psychiatric nurse practitioners may be able to offer somewhat longer follow-up sessions, or be more readily available for consultation than your average psychiatrist.

In an ideal world, your psychiatrist would have expertise in PCOS, but I have yet to find someone with that set of qualifications, so you will likely find yourself educating your doctor about your PCOS.

Pharmacists are a necessity for almost every woman with PCOS, because you are likely to have at least one prescription medication on your must-take list. But many PCOS patients have other conditions unrelated to PCOS that may require medication, and the list can get overwhelming. Where possible (and I know, sometimes you really do have to split things between pharmacies, particularly if you have access to a mail-order pharmacy through your insurance, where cost savings may be quite meaningful), have one pharmacy you deal with consistently. It can be a neighborhood pharmacy, or a big chain store like a CVS, Walgreens, or Rite Aid. Choose one that's convenient geographically, and in terms of its hours. Like most things in life, the easier you make this on yourself, the easier it is to stay in compliance with your medication regime.

An estimated 75% of adults fail to take their medications consistently or properly, thus depriving themselves of the benefits of those medications. Do what you can to end up on the other side of that statistic. If you can identify a particular pharmacist who is there regularly filling your prescriptions and offering the required counseling, take advantage of the opportunity to build a relationship. Also, even if you're doing maintenance prescriptions (those you know for sure you're going to pretty much need forever, so it pays to get them in bulk, like Synthroid) via mail order, take your other prescriptions to the same pharmacy. For example, a new birth control pill or antidepressant, emergency scripts (antibiotics, painkillers), and so on. It may be easy to just go to the pharmacy in your doctor's medical building, but if you've got two prescriptions there, and six at another pharmacy, unless you're being a particularly diligent consumer, it's better to take a few extra minutes and fill it in your standard place, where they've already got all your information.

Relationships are key. If the pharmacist knows you personally or knows a little about you, they're much likelier to give you special attention when you need it. Having an authentic relationship with your pharmacist may offer advantages like:

- Free phone consultations by the pharmacist, not an assistant
- Longer consultations
- Small quantities of a medication to tide you over if they can't reach your doctor quickly when you need a refill
- Extra diligence in following up with your doctor's office regarding refills.

Acupuncturists are licensed practitioners of Traditional Oriental Medicine (Chinese medicine), an ancient system of health care that has been shown to be highly effective for certain conditions, including infertility, stress reduction, and pain management. If your insurance does not cover the services of an acupuncturist, you may want to search for acupuncture schools in your area, which offer services by closely supervised interns at a low fee at their community clinics. Acupuncturists often provide dietary advice, and may prescribe, prepare and dispense medicinal herbs as well. Many people state that they are afraid of needles, or pain, but the needles are very thin, fine needles, and proper insertion is almost painless. The needles are sterile and disposable. The benefits may be huge, so please don't dismiss this option entirely if your first response is fear.

Dentists take care of your teeth, mouth, and gums. Are you wondering why the dentist is on this list? Is PCOS in your mouth? Well, yes and no. Again, because of an increased risk of cardiac problems in women with PCOS, seeing the dentist regularly for preventive care is important. Numerous studies have shown that poor oral hygiene contributes to plaque build-up in the heart – plaque in the mouth, plaque in the heart. See the dentist twice a year for a cleaning, oral cancer screening, etc.

Ophthalmologists are eye doctors. For general eye health and functioning, you should get your eyes checked every year. This is even more important if you've got insulin resistance, pre-diabetes, or diabetes. Over time, elevated blood sugars can contribute to deterioration of the small blood vessels of the body. This causes or contributes to painful conditions such as diabetic neuropathy (loss of sensation in the extremities) and other debilitating conditions such as blindness, diabetic retinopathy (damage to the small blood vessels of the eyes which may cause visual impairment), and even deafness. An ophthalmologist will look at the inside of your eyes quite closely, conduct some painless in-office tests, and be able to detect and treat damage before it can advance. They also treat diseases of the eye, dry eye, and infections, and prescribe and fit contact lenses and glasses.

Plastic Surgeons are MDs who have specialized training in the repair, replacement, or reconstruction of the face and body. Many women with PCOS have one or more body parts that they hate. Sometimes the body part is a problem, and sometimes it's just an unhealthy fixation. I am a strong believer in fixing what you can through natural means such as diet and exercise, but there are some things you just can't fix on your own – abnormal fat deposits, uneven breasts, or a particularly prominent nose. I don't think it's a good idea to go into plastic surgery thinking it's going to fix all your problems, but if you have realistic expectations about a procedure, it can be a huge ego boost. I see the best responses from people who have had breast reduction surgery, tightening of loose neck skin, and tummy tucks (abdominoplasty). You should definitely erase all fantasies of "curing" a weight problem through plastic surgery, especially that pesky abdominal fat. It won't improve your health (sadly!) and, if your weight tends to fluctuate a lot, you will lose the benefit of the surgery quickly. It is extra important to carefully research your plastic surgeon's qualifications. Because these procedures are rarely covered by insurance, it is financially attractive to doctors who may not have a full skill set or true specialization in plastic surgery.

Other Helpful Experts

In addition to the licensed medical professionals I've described above, there are a few more experts it would be nice to have as part of your PCOS care team. These experts are typically certified or, in some cases, such as massage therapists, they may have a local license.

Personal trainer. If you are unsure of what kind of physical fitness program to pursue, have trouble remembering correct form, or need motivation in the form of accountability, then a personal trainer may be helpful. Personal trainers can develop and modify exercise plans that help you achieve your goals for strength training, cardiovascular capacity, and flexibility. Your trainer should be certified – don't just pick the one with the best body! I know it's tempting to just pick the first one you meet, but it behooves you to take a little time, and have a couple of sessions with a trainer to see if his/her training style and attitude mesh with you – you want to feel motivated, not beaten down or shamed. You should feel pushed, but not so exhausted that you lack energy for other activities. Your trainer should be very conscientious about using correct style and methods for weight-lifting and other exercises, in order to prevent injury.

Massage therapist. Because so many women with PCOS report issues with chronic pain, which may be exacerbated by an exercise program, don't avoid exercise, but consider adding an occasional massage to your routine. Massage is available in a range of prices, from low-fee practice sessions at a massage training school, on up to hundreds of dollars for all the bells and whistles at an elite spa. In most urban settings, good massage can be had quite reasonably.

The benefits of massage include relaxation, endorphin release, release of lactic acid build-up in your muscles, and movement of lymph fluid. There are specialized massage therapies available, with styles ranging from gentle to extra-firm. Choose a massage therapist who is certified or, if required by your municipality, licensed. And for really low-budget massage, consider taking a class through your local recreation center, with a friend or spouse/partner, and then trade massages.

Yoga teacher. By now, you know that exercise is good for PCOS. Yoga is a powerful practice. Yoga addresses the physical aspects of strength, balance, and flexibility, and it also addresses the emotional and spiritual components of the mind/body. Yoga teaches acceptance of the body you're in, and where it's at today, moving slowly through change, pushing gently, and other lessons that are particularly critical to PCOS. Yoga practice is accepting of the larger woman, and there are even plus-sized yoga teachers and classes. All postures can be adapted to accommodate your special needs – injuries, an inflexible ankle, etc. As with other practices, there is no one true yoga, but many variations. Before you dismiss yoga, try half a dozen classes with different styles (ashtanga, kundalini, hatha, etc.) and different teachers. Many gyms offer yoga classes as part of the membership, and of course there are private studios. Many of these places will offer a free pass for up to a week, or a special deal on unlimited classes for a month. There are also apps available that allow you to sign up for last-minute classes at different locations, so you don't have to buy a package of classes.

How to Choose a Great Health Care Team Member

You'll notice that I've included a few websites for various professional associations, and these are great places to start getting acquainted with various disciplines, practices, and professions. You don't have to know everything, but I do definitely advise knowing a little bit. A theme you've seen throughout this book is that knowledge is power. You will feel much more empowered when you know what your doctor or other professional is supposed to be doing for you. Although a good doctor will educate you about his or her practice, specialty, and the terms, tests, and procedures you need to know about to get good care, it may take time to build up an experiential knowledge base. Speaking a tiny bit of "their language" is a way to bond more readily with your physician and will help you communicate better. Again, you don't have to know everything – but you should at least know which body part(s) that particular doctor is going to be focusing on before you make the appointment!

The internet is a vast resource, and I am grateful for how easily we can all access information these days. Unfortunately, especially when it comes to medical and health information, it's not always accurate or useful. I won't tell you to limit your searches to critically validated sites like The Mayo Clinic, or well-known resources like WebMD or Dr. Andrew Weil, but I will suggest taking information from other sites with a little skepticism and a critical eye. When you've got PCOS, you're often desperate for both answers and relief. It makes you particularly vulnerable to the seductive claims of clever marketers. Over time, you can evaluate if a particular site is offering a spectrum of thoughtfully gathered information, verifiable results, and the like, or whether they're not offering much specific benefit and seem to mainly be selling you their latest supplement, CD, informational course, or diet plan. Of course, all those things have their place – we all probably need some supplements, dietary counseling is valuable, and other services may be useful as well. But if all the information points in only one direction for the answer, give it a more thorough review. And if it's all bad news, meant to scare you into action, look for the sales pitch there. The news doesn't have to be presented with the neutrality of a Harvard study, but it should be balanced and accurate. There's a tendency to look at every new study as if it's going to be the source of miracles. If there's anything I learned from studying statistics in graduate school, it's that data can be skewed to "prove" just about anything. There is no single answer to the problem of PCOS. Although our symptoms may fall into common categories, each of us has a unique biochemistry, history, and support system that may make a different solution the better choice. There's very rarely a true crisis in PCOS – you should almost always be able to take a little time to study a variety of options, and perhaps consult with another professional.

Consulting with friends is a good way to find a doctor or other professional who meshes with your personality, offers good quality services, and takes your insurance or fits in your price range. Sometimes you have different standards than your friends, but consider it a starting place for a good list of potential candidates.

Referrals from your physician or therapist. I have one physician who seems to hit it right about 95% of the time with her referrals, so I always ask her first. Sometimes she doesn't have anyone to refer me to – but I'd rather that she didn't make a recommendation for someone she doesn't truly believe in. Most doctors are prepared to provide you with a multitude of referrals, and they should be candid in explaining why they're offering that particular referral. Your therapist, particularly if he or she practices Health Psychology as I do, may also be a great resource for referrals. I have a strong network of all of the above types of practitioners and am always meeting with potential additions to my referral list. I believe that the easier it is for you to find a good doctor, the likelier you are to go.

"Best doctor" lists in magazines and newspapers. Many local magazines and newspapers publish annual or periodic lists of "The Best Docs in L.A. County" or "Top 100 Cardiologists," or something similar. Look at these carefully to discern if they're merely paid advertising or "advertorial" type writing. If they are, they're not particularly useful. If they're created by a poll or vote of residents, you may find a doctor who's popular for all the right reasons – or one who's not. A list created through peer review and votes is a much more powerful list and may serve as an excellent starting point if you have no personal referrals. Always do the rest of your homework too, but consider this a pre-screening device. You can easily check various licensing boards to ensure that the provider you're considering has an active license, and no complaints.

Lists in the back of a book. Although these are typically more well-researched and reviewed than other lists, keep in mind the practitioner's personal bias, and their relationships. I've had clients come to me stating that they found a doctor through the lists in a former sitcom star's popular health/diet books. While there may be well-qualified providers on that list, do consider the source. Nonetheless, if you see some of the same names, websites, or titles pop up repeatedly, there's probably a reason, and again, you can start a very good personal search based on someone else's pre-screening.

People you meet on the internet. There are truly amazing resources online for PCOS nowadays, but there are many other PCOS resources popping up with regularity – websites, blogs, referral lists, and Facebook pages. While some of these people may be very sympathetic and informative, please check their credentials thoroughly before taking their advice. Sometimes you may find a golden nugget – the name of the one doctor who really knows something about PCOS.

Websites. There are some excellent websites that offer frequent updates, a sound knowledge base, and a creative and sensitive approach to dealing with PCOS. There's a list of my some of my favorite websites in the Resources section of the book.

Some Additional Cautions

Be cautious with random internet searches and rating sites such as HealthGrades and Yelp! While the advice of your neighbors may point you in the direction of a great restaurant, it's not always the best way to find a doctor or other health care provider. Some practitioners solicit positive reviews from patients or customers by offering discounts or other incentives. These sites are interesting, informative, and entertaining – and you may agree with the reviews you read, but here's where I strongly encourage you to take the information with a grain of salt. It would give me pause to see that an endocrinologist had 15 reviews, and 12 of them were negative for meaningful reasons, like bedside manner or competence – but it's human nature to complain, so reviews are more likely to get posted when they're negative than positive. Most of the time, we just thank someone and go about our business if we're pleased. If we're unhappy, however, the internet offers an infinitely broader audience for our complaints.

Be mindful that many professional organizations charge significant fees to their professional members, which include a listing on the organization's website. Just because a physician or other provider isn't listed on an association's website doesn't mean they're not qualified, but you may have to ask more screening questions. It may mean they don't entirely support the organization's goals, they don't want to spend money on advertising, or they haven't heard of the organization yet. Some organizations have official sounding names that seem impressive, but they aren't respected by the practitioners themselves!

If it seems that I'm serving as more of a consumer advocate than a mental health practitioner in this section, let me explain why. People are often intimidated, fearful, anxious, and overwhelmed when it comes to selecting healthcare providers. Maybe it's your insurance company pressuring you to pick a name from a list of HMO physicians in order to complete your sign-up. Maybe you've just gotten a scary diagnosis and you need help NOW. Maybe it's a spouse or partner who just wants you to take the easy route and go see the family doctor when you really need a specialist. Regardless, it's easy with an incurable condition like PCOS to find yourself lured in by claims of a cure. The worlds of medicine and psychotherapy are competitive businesses, particularly in the larger metropolises. Awareness of sales and marketing techniques, the power of the internet, and the variety of resources at your disposal will serve to empower you as a patient, and I believe that contributes to a better overall outcome.

Managing Your Relationship with Your Doctor

We've been socialized to think that doctors know more than the rest of us and, in certain respects, they do. Nonetheless, you are the expert on your own body. Sure, doctors can run tests, make observations, and apply a depth of knowledge that you may not have but, in the end, you're the only one who has to live in that body. So be respectful, but also command respect by doing your own research, and making thoughtful decisions.

Making Decisions Like a Professional

People in business are called upon to make decisions large and small every day. Politicians, mothers, and people of leisure are too. And women with PCOS have a lot more medical and self-care decisions to make than the average woman. It can all be quite confusing and overwhelming. What separates the good decision makers from the bad decision makers is applying a basic set of principles to the practice of decision-making. These are steps for making decisions you feel good about:

Take a deep breath. Trite but useful is the advice to "take a deep breath first." There's a really good reason for this too – when you tense up, your breathing becomes constricted, stress hormones are released, and your body's energetic resources are directed towards fleeing from danger. Other than "get out of here," evolution has taught your body that the brain doesn't need much clear-thinking ability, but the legs need a lot of glucagon for power. So, your body's primed for action, and your brain is near worthless other than to conduct automatic functions like sustaining heart rate and breathing.

How bad is it? Few things are as intense as we initially perceive them to be. There are notable exceptions, of course – major car crashes, profound birth defects, cancer diagnoses, and the like. But sometimes, what first appears to be a problem may actually be an opportunity, or a blessing:

- Getting fired may mean you have more time to spend with your family, or an opportunity to start the consulting business you've been thinking of opening.
- A diabetes diagnosis may be just the kick-start you need to start a healthier diet and exercise program.
- Your child breaks the house rules - and an antique vase that you never liked much anyway. Your conscience has just been relieved of the guilt of getting rid of Aunt Mary's heirloom.
- Your spouse leaves you for another woman, which gives you a chance to start over and make a better choice in your next relationship.

Our initial tendency is often to catastrophize, meaning create or perceive something as monumental where there's either no problem, or a much milder or less severe problem. This might look like:

- Declaring the evening an unsalvageable wreck when your boyfriend calls to say he's stuck in traffic and you've got dinner reservations at a place that's always booked solid – and it's Friday night. But you didn't really feel like going out anyway, and you end up ordering in and having a cuddle-fest instead, which was better than the noisy chaotic restaurant experience.
- Listing a bunch of small problems (the dog is sick, my glucose was elevated on my last lab results, I've lost some important tickets, my car needs expensive repairs, and my son's school is taking an extra teacher in-service day on short notice) and concluding that your life is a disaster and everything's out of control (note, saying "always" and "never" are good clues that you might be catastrophizing).
- Omitting pertinent details – for example, "my car needs $800 worth of repairs and it's only a year old!" – to elicit attention and

sympathy. The truth gets scaled down substantially when you clarify that a) the car needed regular service anyway; b) some of these issues are still covered under warranty so it will cost you nothing; and c) you have a coupon from the dealer that makes the balance practically free. Big difference from "and it's going to cost nearly a thousand dollars!"

- Do yourself a favor – take the drama out of the problem, and it will make others respect and pay attention to your legitimate needs more readily, help you calm yourself down, and allow you to think from a more centered place when you're not embellishing the details to get attention.

Consider true urgency. Some problems really do need immediate attention. They usually involve blood, the law, and meaningful sums of money. Beyond that, it's all negotiable. Quite often, things that we think require urgent attention (tears, screaming, or ominously thick envelopes from the Internal Revenue Service) need to be handled, but they're not a crisis. Sometimes other people's emotions undo our rational thought processes. And the IRS elevates just about everyone's blood pressure – BUT, there's still time to deal with it. And sometimes, there are things that don't have a deadline and never seem to get done. I've learned that when I don't do something for a really long time, I actually don't WANT to do it. When I get to that realization, I consider whether that is something I should give my attention to at all. Refining your priority list (by refining, I really mean reducing) will naturally lead to a lessened sense of urgency.

Do some research. This used to mean going to the library, maybe talking to a few friends or your doctor or spouse. Nowadays, we interpret it to mean scouring the internet for hours and reading everything you can get our hands on, until it's two in the morning, your eyes can't focus on anything further away than the monitor, and you're confused beyond belief. The internet is a gift – use it wisely. Identify a couple of people in your life who really are generally reliable, trustworthy, thoughtful, and sensible. They may be teachers, neighbors, a parent or spouse, a friend who works in the medical field, or a member of your church or temple. Use them to review and discuss what you learn from your doctors, and from the internet. It helps if this advisor is not prone to drama, and not easily sucked in by hype. If you tend to be enticed by claims of easy success, or "expertise" that's nothing more than unsupported opinion, it's valuable to have an ally or two who will remind you of what actually makes sense.

Case Example, Elaine:

> Elaine was desperate for some relief from her PMS symptoms, and the never-ending growth of unwelcome facial hair. She'd tried birth control pills, Spironolactone, homeopathic cures, and acupuncture. Her yoga teacher, Suzanna, was going to India and suggested that she consult with someone there. Elaine was very excited, because she knew Ayurveda was an ancient system of healing and surely, they would have some answers. Suzanna brought back half a suitcase full of foul-smelling, strange looking pills and liquids for Elaine. Elaine consulted with a doctor friend of hers who (not so gently) said: "Elaine, you won't eat anything except organic food; why on earth would you consume herbs you don't even know the name of, from a country that has marginal sanitation at best? That's crazy!" Okay, maybe not so gentle, but it certainly was exactly what Elaine needed to hear before taking treatments that were not necessarily either safe or suitable for her condition. Elaine allowed herself to slow down, consult with a known and trusted expert and friend, and was willing to take well-reasoned advice. This is smart decision making.

Case Example, Uma:

> Uma had been diagnosed with allergies to tree nuts (walnuts, almonds, etc.), avocadoes, and pineapple. But she was desperate to lose some weight, so she had a

consultation with the clerk at her neighborhood health food story. The clerk had written a little book about diet, so Uma figured she must know a thing or two. She insisted that, if Uma followed a healthful, raw, cleansing diet, consisting mainly of salads, raw vegetables and fruits, nuts, and avocadoes, her body would recover, allergies would be a thing of the past, and Uma would be the picture of health. Uma bravely tried, although she was worried when her mouth started swelling after eating the nuts. Uma was also nauseous and lacked energy after every meal. The clerk told her that she was "detoxing." Uma persisted until she became very sick and began breaking out in hives, at which point she went to the doctor. In fact, Uma had essentially been poisoning herself with this seemingly-healthy raw foods diet – because she couldn't tolerate some of the primary ingredients! Uma was really lucky she didn't end up in anaphylactic shock, a potentially fatal reaction to extreme nut allergy.

Medical Records

In addition to finding the right medical professionals to help, you're going to need to keep track of what you're currently doing, and what you've tried in the past. Good record keeping is essential to living well with PCOS.

Here are five tips to help you:

1. Get a copy of all your labs and make your own medical file – paper or digital, whatever works for you.
2. Keep a running list of surgeries or procedures, because you WILL eventually forget the dates and even the doctors.

3. Type up and print out a list of your medications to hand to new doctors. Include a list of herbs and supplements.

4. Keep a list of your drug allergies, if any, in your phone, as well as on a written record you give to your doctors.

5. Have all your doctors copied on your lab work – it's a push of a button for the lab, typically, and will save you a lot of checking and photocopying.

Also send these documents to yourself via e-mail and drop them into a file devoted exclusively to medical information. I can't tell you how many times a lab report hasn't made its way to the doctor. Rather than wasting the appointment time, I've pulled up the record on my phone and handed it to the doctor. This benefits you as well as your doctor.

CHAPTER 9

Food Essentials for Mental Health

F ar from being the exclusive purview of dieticians and other weight-loss experts, diet is inextricably linked with PCOS and the mental health issues that accompany it. Along with quality sleep, appropriate medical care, prescription medication, supplementation, exercise, and meditation, eating well is one of the pillars of good mental health. If you're surviving on junk food, processed food, fast food, empty calories, or too many refined carbs and not enough protein or good fats, you are going to be wildly deficient in necessary nutrients and amino acids that fuel the brain. Without those good ingredients going into your body, you simply don't have enough energy, the building blocks for your neurotransmitters, or the ability to lose PCOS-related weight.

This chapter addresses some of the more common problematic foods and eating behaviors, the healthier and optimal choices, and some steps for making the transition from one end of that spectrum to the other, with particulars on how certain foods and nutrients feed or distress your brain. It is meant to get you started on the necessary changes that contribute to good mental health.

Problematic Foods/Behaviors for PCOS Brain Health

While diet isn't the entire reason you feel bad, it's potentially a big part of the reason. Diet can contribute to a depleted supply of the building blocks your neurotransmitters need to make you happy, hypoglycemia that leads to mood swings, hormonal irregularities (remember, your brain is bathed in hormones too), and eating disorders. Eating the wrong diet can lead to:

- Inadequate consumption of essential fatty acids, which are derived from protein sources.
- Ignoring the role of your thyroid, which may be causing unnecessary weight gain, as well as slowing your metabolism, which makes weight loss harder.
- Eating too many of the wrong calories.

Drinking your calories. I'm talking juice, soda, mixed drinks, beer, energy drinks, sweet tea, ice blended coffee drinks, mochas, lattes, chai, and even milk. It's okay to drink some of them, but if you're always sipping on something caloric, you're taking in a lot of unnecessary calories, which limits your desire or ability to consume healthy things that contribute to brain health.

The white stuff. I'm definitely talking about sugar here, but also other refined carbohydrates like white bread, pasta, white rice, many milks, French fries, crackers, potato chips, and the like. White foods like egg whites, cauliflower, and unsweetened Greek yogurt are better white foods. Generally, the less color a food has, the less nutrient density (iceberg lettuce vs. kale, white potatoes vs. yams, etc.).

Poor quality proteins. Anything processed beyond recognition, designed to simulate a real food (processed cheese food – YUK!), fast food burgers or chicken, lunch meat, and proteins from most restaurants (if they don't specify free-range, organic, or grass-fed, they're probably not particularly healthy). As a rule, the cheaper it is, the likelier it is to be low quality.

Wheat. I'm not going to tell you that you must be gluten-free or else. I do have a strong preference for organic wheat products over conventionally farmed wheat. Organic wheat is free of the herbicide glyphosate - a potent chemical, endocrine disrupter, and neurotoxin. Enough said. Is a little every now and then going to kill you? No. But avoid it as much as reasonably possible, even when it's a little awkward or inconvenient.

Dairy. This is another much-discussed PCOS dietetics issue. As children, most of us were taught that two to four servings a day of dairy foods were key to good health; we now know that this is not the case. As it relates to brain health, there's the very real factor of something called casomorphin - protein fragments derived from the milk protein casein, which have an opioid effect. So, if you're one of those people who says: "I could give it all up ... except cheese ... NO WAY!" you may have a legitimate addiction to the opioid effects of dairy.

Many people recommend banning all forms of dairy absolutely, based on their potential as endocrine disrupters affecting estrogen and insulin regulation, their high fat content and potential contamination. The reality is, you can live without dairy. If you have a casein allergy, are lactose intolerant, or are trying to conceive, it may be one of those controllable factors you want to consider. Or, you may be able to tolerate a little GI discomfort or other side effects to have the dairy products you love. Consider your personal situation.

Soy is a bean that is consumed as human and animal food worldwide. It is another food that is the subject of much disagreement in the PCOS world, due to its estrogenic effects. It is a phytoestrogen, which means that it weakly mimics the actions of estrogen. On the plus side, it can be very helpful for heart disease, cancer prevention, and symptoms of menopause. For PCOS specifically, it may help reduce testosterone, insulin, cholesterol, and inflammatory markers.

I'm with the group that generally considers soy unhealthy in processed form, such as the ubiquitous soybean oil, soy protein powders, meat alternatives, and soymilk. "Bad soy" is found in abundance in processed foods like granola bars, protein bars, protein pastas, and even foods promoted as healthy vegetarian alternatives. Traditional fermented forms of soy, such as natto, miso, tempeh, soy sauce, and fermented tofu or soymilk are fine. Again, you have to consider your own body and preferences. If you are vegan or vegetarian, it may be an important source of both protein and calories, and I don't believe in unnecessarily limiting one's diet.

Other allergens. Although many people say they have allergies, very few people have a true food allergy resulting in a breathing emergency called anaphylactic shock. Many of us, however, have food sensitivities. The following account for about 90% of food allergies: milk, eggs, peanuts, tree nuts (like walnuts, pecans, almonds), soy, wheat and other gluten-containing grains (barley, rye, oats), fish, and shellfish. First, notice that a lot of the foods I've already mentioned as potentially problematic for PCOS patients are on the allergen list. Basically, if you're allergic to or sensitive to foods, but continue to consume them anyway, you're contributing to inflammation in your body and brain.

Diet/artificial sweeteners. I grew up thinking soda was a treat, and seeing the skinny ladies drinking Tab and Fresca. Naturally, since I wanted to be thin too, I thought diet soda was the way to go, along with diet sweetener laced coffee and treats. "Free calories!" Well, not really. I'm vehemently opposed to all artificial sweeteners. I don't care what's allegedly safe or not; there are too many potential side effects of these chemicals on your brain. They also skew appetite sensors, activate insulin (so you might as well eat real sugar), and can cause headaches and gastrointestinal distress. Better to eat a little of the real stuff and train your taste buds to look for less sweet tastes.

Not eating enough calories. This flies in the face of conventional wisdom, but bear with me for a moment. When you don't eat enough (and "enough" is probably far more than you'd think), your metabolism slows down to a snail's crawl, and your body holds on, subconsciously fearing impending starvation. "Bonus" – you get food cravings, headaches, irritability, mood swings, blood sugar drops, fatigue, and lethargy! Find a good online calculator to determine your number, or work with a dietician.

Not nearly enough fruits and vegetables. Food cravings are a constant complaint of women with PCOS, often leading to food binges, and feelings of shame and self-loathing. The best cure is eating enough protein, eating regularly, and eating plenty of produce, mainly vegetables. Eating all the vegetables means that your micronutrient needs are met and remarkably, cravings tend to disappear. Produce is also full of fiber, low in calories, and easier on the planet than meat, dairy, and grain.

Jumping headfirst into every dietary trend/fad. Weight and health management are challenging topics. There are innumerable new eating plans and diets coming out every year, all competing for attention with extravagant promises. Some of the more popular ones in the last few years include the auto-immune protocol, the thyroid diet, gluten-free, Paleo ("the caveman diet"), vegan, the Master Cleanse, the alkaline diet, candida diet, ketogenic diets, the blood type diet, the baby food diet, the grapefruit diet, intermittent fasting, the cabbage soup diet, and the HCG protocol. And those are just the ones I can think of off the top of my head.

Many of them are alluring for women with PCOS because they promise not only weight loss, but relief from fatigue, aching joints, menstrual irregularity, and so much more. Anything that calls for you to eliminate entire food groups for lengthy periods of time, or requires elaborate testing, planning, and coordination, is going to be really hard to stick with. "Results may vary" is a term that we don't seem to take too seriously when embarking on the next dietary trend. In the end, you know the real answer is moderation, even though that's not trendy. It's true that our nutritional information can change over time, but be aware of what is fact and what is fiction.

Any disordered eating behavior. Women with PCOS already have a much, much higher rate of eating disorders than women without PCOS. Going on a diet often triggers those behaviors or contributes to the maintenance of a pre-existing eating disorder. Engaging in eating disordered behavior usually involves under eating or overeating and purging, using exercise excessively, or other unhealthy behaviors. There may be some short-term payoff, but the long-term side effects are a constant weight, a further disturbed metabolism, dental and esophageal damage, heart and kidney damage, dehydration, fatigue, hair loss, and so much more. If you have an eating disorder, or think you have an eating disorder, please seek help from a therapist who is an eating disorder professional.

Better Food Choices and Behaviors for PCOS Brain Health

Food Habits

Eat protein. Protein is needed for optimal amino acid balance. This is an enormous subject, and there are book suggestions for further reading in the Resources section of this book. When the body lacks essential amino acids, which are necessary for your neurotransmitters to work properly, your mental health suffers. The reasons for this problem may be under-consuming protein, inadequate absorption of the protein you do consume due to gut issues, or the wrong mix of available amino acids. If you suspect this may be a problem for you, it's worth doing some research. Consider taking a targeted amino acid supplement to see if that helps; there are nutritionists who are trained in this protocol.

Here's a guideline for how much protein you need. One ounce of protein is about seven grams of protein, and we want to get 20 – 30 grams (three to four ounces) of protein per meal, and around 10 grams of protein per snack. If you eat snacks, you can eat toward the lower end of the meal protein requirement (more like three ounces than four); otherwise, stay toward the higher end.

I've included some of the more common sources of protein below, along with average servings and what that might look like for our purposes. I recommend getting comfortable with what an ounce, two ounces, half a cup, etc. looks like by weighing, measuring, checking package labels, or using a tool like MyFitnessPal.com just until you get the idea, and then stop. Too much obsessing over calories and other details often contributes to disordered eating behavior, and it's tedious. The whole point of eating like this is to calm down, eat peacefully, and enjoy your healthy food and lifestyle.

Protein Source	Snack Serving	Meal Serving
Protein powder	1 – 2 scoops	2 – 3 scoops
Milk	1 cup	
Greek yogurt	½ cup plain	1 full cup

Eggs	1 egg	2 – 3 eggs
Peanut butter	2 Tbsp.	
Nuts	1 oz	
Chicken	1 – 2 oz	4 – 5 oz
Beef/pork	1 – 2 oz	3 – 4 oz
Lamb chops	1 "lollipop" chop	1 medium chop
Sunflower seeds	¼ cup	
Cottage Cheese	½ cup	1 cup
Fish	2 oz	4 – 6 oz
Shellfish/shrimp	2 oz	6 oz (12 – 18 large shrimp)
Cheese	1 oz	3 oz
Beans/lentils	½ cup	1 cup
Tofu (soybean curd)	½ cup	1 cup

Eat a substantial breakfast (around 500 – 700 calories, or about one quarter to one third of your daily calories, depending upon whether you snack or not). I know breakfast is really hard for a lot of women with PCOS or insulin resistance, so start out by drinking it if you must, and then start integrating solid foods that provide better satiety.

Here's my favorite smoothie recipe (note that it is NOT loaded up with fruit; the commercially made smoothies you may be used to can contain over 90 grams of carbohydrates in the form of pure, fast-acting fruit sugars). They may taste great, but they are NOT healthy. They will destabilize your blood sugar and leave you a mess for the rest of the day.

Dr. Gretchen's Smoothie Recipe
8 oz unsweetened organic rice, almond, or coconut milk
1 – 2 scoops of raw brown rice or pea protein powder or ¼ cup chia seeds
2/3 cup frozen organic berries or other fruit
A tablespoon of coconut oil, olive oil, or 1/8 avocado
A little sweetener if needed
A dash of vanilla extract if desired
A hearty shake of cinnamon

I like to add all flavors of berries or peaches to vanilla protein powder for Berries 'n' Cream, Peaches 'n' Cream, etc. Chocolate protein powder is great with strawberries, raspberries, or a spoonful of peanut butter (even better, try organic peanut butter powder, which is defatted, mixes easily, and has all of the flavor!) or almond butter. I'm allergic to bananas, so I don't use them, but if you do, limit it to half a banana.

Some of my other favorite easy, high-protein (note: cheese may be non-dairy/vegan cheeses) breakfasts include:

- One cup of plain whole milk Greek yogurt with half a cup of fresh sliced berries and a handful of nuts. Skip granola; it's one of the biggest junk foods masquerading as health food.
- Two hardboiled eggs (unpeeled, these last for a few days in the refrigerator) and two pieces of fruit or one slice of buttered whole grain bread or gluten-free bread and one piece of fruit.
- Real buckwheat crepes with a handful of berries. Made over the weekend, these can be stored in the refrigerator for up to a week. Buckwheat is not a grain; it's the seed of a flowering fruit. With a little practice, these crepes are easy to make, and leftovers can also be filled with savory ingredients like scrambled eggs, cheese, chopped up poultry or ham, cooked vegetables, etc. for a light but satisfying meal.
- Scrambled eggs with cheese, avocado slices, sour cream, and a lot of salsa, along with half a cup of refried or whole beans.
- An omelet with as many vegetables (leftover from the previous day or two's meals) stuffed in it as possible, held together with a little cheese if you'd like, and topped with salsa.
- Leftovers of any sort. Just because we think of breakfast foods as looking like eggs or cereal doesn't mean you can't eat rice, tofu, fish, homemade lasagna or meatloaf, a hamburger, or any other food you enjoy. Experiment and see what works for you.

Forget counting calories or grams of anything after you've learned the basics. Use the plate method, with your plate made up of half leafy green/low-carbohydrate vegetables, a quarter protein, and a quarter carbohydrates, with some high-quality fat thrown in for good measure.

Eat unlimited produce. Low-carb vegetables include:

- Bean sprouts
- Red, yellow, orange, and green bell peppers
- Chives, green onions, shallots, onion, garlic
- Eggplant
- Spinach
- Chard, kale, and other dark leafy greens
- Tomatoes
- Cucumbers
- Radishes
- Lettuce
- Cabbage
- Cauliflower
- Artichokes
- Green chilies
- Carrots
- Jicama
- Sprouts of all kinds
- Snow peas
- Bok choy
- Mushrooms
- Green beans
- Broccoli
- Asparagus
- Zucchini
- Leeks
- Parsley
- Celery

Easy Ways to Increase Vegetable Consumption

Not everyone loves vegetables. Some of us downright loathe them. But the reality is, you cannot meet your nutritional needs without eating a lot of vegetables, every single day. A word about juicing: I'm against it, unless it's pure green juice (like celery, parsley, lemon, cucumber, lettuce mix), and even then, only in very small quantities. I don't think relying on juice as a primary source of nutrients is wise. Besides, it's expensive and often inconvenient, and you can't always get the organic produce you should ideally be choosing. Here are some easy ways to consistently eat your veggies:

Sautéed mix. A stir-fry is the classic, but any compatible mix of vegetables, made in some quantity and stored for a few days, will make the task easier. I like mushrooms, onions, and a variety of bell peppers sautéed together. For variety, add fresh tomatoes. This is great served with eggs, chicken, tofu, or fish.

Salad. The other classic source of vegetables. I'm of mixed mind in the raw versus cooked vegetable debate, siding with more cooked vegetables for those with sensitive tummies/gut issues, and advocating for fresh, raw, organic vegetables to tolerance. Make it big, brightly colored, diverse, and with an oil/vinegar dressing instead of some creamy, processed, thick commercially prepared stuff. Turn it into a meal with leftover beans, chicken, shrimp, steak, a little cheese, chopped up hardboiled eggs, etc.

One-vegetable soup. This is one of my favorite preparations. It makes consuming lots of vegetables so easy. Take any of the following vegetables: carrot, broccoli, cauliflower, mushroom, onion, zucchini, or tomato. Cook up about two cups of it, until soft, in a little olive oil, with salt, pepper, and any other desired spices (the cauliflower is excellent with some curry powder and turmeric in it). Whirl in a high-speed blender (like a Ninja) with about two cups of chicken stock or homemade bone broth. Adjust the seasoning to taste, adding a little organic heavy cream or coconut milk if you want a creamier soup. Garnish with a drizzle of olive oil or a bit of ghee and eat about half of it. Share the other half with a friend, or save it for tomorrow, and take it to work in a tightly sealed mason jar, which can be used for direct reheating.

Eat salad for breakfast. Just be sure to include a generous amount of protein. Leftover cooked vegetables in an omelet or as a side with eggs are excellent. You could even do a hearty serving of vegetable soup with beans in it, for a one-bowl meal.

Substitute an extra vegetable for the rice/potato/pasta side at a restaurant. I had a friend who hated vegetables. We'd go out to eat and he'd ask the waiter to substitute another starch for the dreaded vegetables (so he'd be eating steak with rice AND potatoes, or pork spareribs with corn AND macaroni salad). I want you to do the opposite: identify at least one, if not two, starches and ask for them to be substituted with vegetables. Some places will offer as little as a lousy side of lettuce and tomatoes that serve as hamburger toppings. Others will give you a generous steamed or sautéed side of mixed vegetables. Even a side salad is great. The goal is to end up with at least two vegetable servings.

Hack your sandwich. Sometimes the only thing available is a sandwich. Ask for it to be prepared open-faced (without the bread on top), or remove the top bread yourself. Ask to load it up with double vegetables; this is a particularly great strategy at submarine sandwich places. Have your sandwich toppings dumped in a bowl with a bunch of lettuce or spinach. Try to get a little side salad (even at places like this that don't offer salads as a menu item, you might be able to get them to construct a little "salad" out of the fixings, and they typically have vinegar and oil available as sandwich toppings).

Snack on vegetables. Carrots, celery, jicama, and other raw vegetables all lend themselves to easy snacking, and are great as long as you're not loading them up with blue cheese dressing. Celery with peanut butter or hummus with carrot sticks are classic snacks that are good for you, as long as you're mindful not to over consume the peanut butter or hummus.

Make "meatless Monday" a habit, along with at least one other day per week. Many people prefer not to give up meat permanently, but want to contribute to the health of the planet by going vegan or vegetarian one day per week. This gave rise to the "Meatless Monday" movement. By giving up meat 15% of the time (one day a week), you improve health risk factors, reduce consumption of water and fossil fuels, and decrease your carbon footprint. Not coincidentally, it means you're going to have to eat more vegetables!

Substitute vegetables for rice. Instead of ordering a rice bowl, get a veggie bowl with a small side of brown rice. This trick works at all the "fresh Mex" places like Chipotle, when ordering sushi/sashimi bowls to go, and at Chinese restaurants. Basically, instead of letting the restaurant load up two thirds of your bowl with rice, you're going to ask for steamed/sautéed/stir-fried/raw vegetables, and then do your protein and toppings as usual. It's often quite a bit tastier than a bowl of bland starch too.

Order fajitas instead of something fried at a Mexican restaurant. Yes, it's possible to eat relatively healthy food at a Mexican restaurant. Send the chips back and skip the queso appetizer. Ignore anything deep-fried. Eat the fajitas without the tortillas, but go ahead and have a small serving of beans. Order shrimp or fish "al mojo de ajo" (with garlic). Get chicken, fish, or meatball (albondigas) soup. Eat the guacamole because it's a healthy fat.

Choose Asian restaurants more often, including East Indian. Most Asian cuisines rely heavily on vegetables, and they often have a huge variety of flavors, spices, and colors. The proportion of vegetables to protein is usually far better than you'll find with typical Western food, although you do have to carefully monitor your consumption of rice or noodles. Indian food is one of the best ways to get both amazingly flavorful vegetables and a dose of healthy anti-inflammatory spices like turmeric and ginger. Just don't eat too much *naan*!

Learn how to order from the "secondi" and sides at Italian restaurants. Along with Mexican food, the perception is that you just can't eat healthy food at an Italian restaurant, and that is simply not true. Many pasta-oriented restaurants are now offering gluten-free options. By skipping the entrée pastas and ordering from the "secondi" – the meat, fish, and chicken dishes – you will be able to stay healthy and balanced. There are many nice salads, sautéed spinach, and other cooked vegetables. If your protein comes with a tiny side of pasta, as it often does, that's fine to eat. Just ignore the fluffy Italian bread that comes with everything, and you should be in good shape. As a bonus, you won't have a carb hangover like everyone else in your party.

Eat healthy fats and avoid hydrogenated or partially hydrogenated fats. Healthy fats include olive oil, coconut oil, grass-fed butter, nuts and nut oils, and avocados. The fat in fish and grass-fed meat is also considered healthy fat. Avoid junk fats, like corn, soy, and safflower oils, most margarines, and shortening. These are commonly found in processed foods, like pastries and salad dressings. Simply by avoiding the bad fats, you will eliminate loads of fats that you shouldn't be eating anyway. The fat of factory-farmed animals is also unhealthy. Avoid eating oxidized fats (including nuts) – ones that smell rancid – as well.

More Food Specifics and Tips for Handling Food Challenges

Eating shouldn't be as complicated as it usually is now. I'm a big advocate for simplicity and sustainability. Here are some things to keep in mind as you start reforming your diet to enhance your brain health.

Start by increasing your protein at every meal/snack. I can't emphasize the importance of protein and brain health enough, so I'll tell you again: you need plenty of it to ensure brain health. *The amino acids that fuel your neurotransmitters and make you feel good come from protein.* You also need a decent amount of protein to satisfy your appetite, especially when you're cutting down on carbohydrates. What is enough? Two to three ounces at breakfast, and four to six ounces (depending upon hunger) at each of lunch and dinner will do it. There's no need to supplement with protein powders or bars. Real, whole food will be the most satisfying as well as the most nutritious, but if you really struggle with breakfast, I'm all for a good quality protein powder supplement used to form a palatable, low-sugar smoothie.

Add the vegetables you love in greater quantity. Quite often, these are the higher carb ones, which include things we think of as quite obviously vegetables, and some that tend to get categorized as grains or legumes (but they really are technically fruits):

- **Corn** is the subject of much debate. It is known to be highly allergenic, frequently genetically modified, and of course, it is used to fatten up cattle. That's not a great recommendation! However, corn is also one of the staple foods of many cultures, gluten-free, and high in fiber and phytonutrients. It's also tasty and inexpensive. If you always aim for organic corn products, and don't overindulge, it can definitely be part of a healthy diet.

- **Yams/sweet potatoes**. Substituting yams or sweet potatoes for regular old white potatoes is often recommended because they are more nutrient dense. They are a good source of healthy carbs, can be easily prepared in many ways, and provide necessary variety. When people make major dietary changes, including cutting all the starchy carbs, I often see them experience lethargy and more brain fog. Adding back in just a small portion – say, half a medium baked yam – of healthy carbs can restore a lot of your energy.

- **Red and golden beets** are delicious cold or hot, and make a great salad with some goat cheese, pistachios, and dark greens.

- **Parsnips/rutabaga/turnips.** I lump these all together because they appear fresh around the same time of year and make great hearty and healthy soups, or a substantial side dish when baked or roasted.

- **Winter squash** also tend to appear in clusters in the late fall, and are delicious roasted in the oven, just brushed with a little olive oil and topped with sea salt.

- **Peas** are high in protein, as well as fiber. They are considered to be one of the most hypoallergenic proteins, which is why pea protein powder is often recommended, especially for women with PCOS. I prefer to eat my peas whole and fresh, as a solo item or mixed in with other foods, but will resort to pea protein occasionally.

- **Cooked onions** have a distinctive sweetness and can be caramelized for richness. They're a delicious topping for meats, with other vegetables, or in a soup.

- **Yucca/cassava** are not the same, but are often confused, and share many similarities. They are commonly found in the diets of many cultures around the world, but not often in western culture. Cassava root flour is an excellent substitute for wheat flour if you are following a gluten-free diet.
- **Beans** of all types are high fiber and a good source of protein. They are cheap, readily available, and adaptable. More importantly, beans contain resistant starch (the opposite of the digestible starch that tends to increase blood sugar), which helps feed the healthy bacteria in your gut, which helps you digest and absorb nutrients, and ultimately, supports brain health. Pretty big benefits from the humble bean!
- **Quinoa** is one of the ancient grains that has become quite trendy. It is a complete protein, containing all the essential amino acids that are necessary for neurotransmitter health. It's fairly versatile as well, serving as a side dish, a salad, or made into meatless patties.
- **Legumes/pulses** include soy, peanuts, lentils, and chickpeas (as well as fresh and dried peas and other beans). These foods are nicely balanced in terms of protein, carbohydrate, and fat. Chickpeas (garbanzo beans) contain d-chiro-inositol, which is helpful for women with PCOS. Soy and peanuts are common allergens, however, so you should be mindful of your own tolerance or intolerance.

Add the vegetables and fruits you like less until you hit at least two cups per day. Four cups per day of the colorful, low carb ones (basically, everything not listed above) is even better, but I'm realistic. If this sounds like a lot, start with a cup and increase the volume as you get more accustomed to shifting your diet toward vegetables.

Choose only **healthy fats**, and consume about three tablespoons per day. Note that this is about triple what dieters commonly consume. Your brain needs fat for optimal functioning. In fact, your brain is made up of about 60% fat! Essential fatty acids are critical for proper functioning.

Healthy fats increase satiety (the sense of being full) and help decrease food cravings. The following are among the best healthy sources of fat:

- **Grass-fed butter** – butter from grass-fed cows is higher in Omega-3 fatty acids and vitamin K2 than butter from grain-fed cows. It also is five times higher in CLA (conjugated linoleic acid), a popular weight-loss supplement.
- **Ghee** is clarified butter (heated to separate the milk solids, which also happens to make it highly tolerable for most people, even those with a sensitivity to dairy). It is commonly used in Indian cooking, and has a higher burn point, so it is a versatile fat.
- **Olive oil** is high in oleic acid, one of the fatty acids. It is highly anti-inflammatory, as well as containing antioxidants. A common feature of the Mediterranean diet, it is reputed to improve depression and decrease dementia rates.
- **Coconut oil** contains medium chain fatty acids (MCFAs). When digested, it creates ketones which are easily accessed by the brain for energy. It is anti-inflammatory, antifungal, and antibacterial. The MCFAs help balance insulin in your cells, which is a major bonus.
- **Avocado** also benefits brain function and may lower cholesterol levels. It's delicious as guacamole, sliced on toast, in a salad, or eaten out of hand with a little balsamic vinegar. Avocado oil is also readily available and makes a nice substitute for olive oil if you don't like the flavor of it.
- **Wild caught fish** that is high in Omega-3s (anchovies, sardines, salmon, Bluefin tuna, Pacific halibut, and rainbow trout, among others) is good for memory and brain health.
- **Grass-fed meats** are healthy fat sources for the same reasons as grass-fed butter.

A Caution About Fats

Never eat a fat, oil, or predominantly fatty food that smells rancid. Rancid fats are very unhealthy. Also, despite what you may have heard about it not being possible to eat too much fat, it absolutely IS possible to eat too much fat. Even when you're on a carb-restricted diet, calories do matter. This is an area where women with PCOS may have a problem, because if your brain isn't balanced yet, you're still going to have the cravings and feel hungry, regardless of how much fat you eat.

Other Tips and Tricks

If you're still hungry after eating all the vegetables, healthy proteins, and healthy fats, **then** eat some healthy carbs that are whole foods. You might be surprised to find that you don't even want them, or you want very little. It doesn't take long for your brain and your body to adapt to this healthier fuel and support you by rejecting the unhealthier foods.

Learn the art of assemblage or "non-cooking cooking." A lot of women tell me they can't cook, or cooking is complicated, or takes too much time. I get it. Life is busy, and time is short. When you can't cook, you need to come up with meals that are virtually as healthy as homemade foods. Luckily, with the breadth of prepared foods available at supermarkets, you should have no problem sourcing:

- Healthy proteins like roasted chicken, cooked salmon filets, cooked shrimp, hand-carved lean roast beef or turkey, cheeses of all sorts, canned sardines and tuna, nut butters, and cooked and peeled hardboiled eggs.
- Vegetables of every variety. Take some time to scout out a well-stocked salad bar. You can source the ingredients for an extremely colorful and nutritious salad, pick out some cooked items, or use the cut and washed vegetables to make a stir fry or other dish at home quickly and easily. "Salad in a bag" becomes "meal in a bag" when you add a handful of chopped chicken, turkey,

or egg. Frozen vegetables are another great resource. They are easy to store and use in small portions. There are also prepared frozen vegetable dishes that can add some variety to your diet, like spinach patties, vegetable soufflé, etc.

- Fruits, of course. Buy small quantities of the easily perishable things, like raspberries, and larger quantities of old standbys that last a while when refrigerated, like apples and oranges. Generally, avoid dried fruits, because they're basically candy in natural form.

- Frozen foods and meals are all over the place in terms of quality, and they tend to have way too many carbs for women with PCOS, but there are some that are suitable. Look for vegetarian, organic, and vegetable-heavy ethnic foods. Learn to read the labels enough that you can get the right ratio of carbohydrates and protein for your needs. I aim for at least 25 grams of protein (about 3½ ounces worth) and no more than 30 – 35 grams of carbohydrate (the equivalent of about two slices of bread or an ear of corn). Poor choices typically include pasta dishes, burritos, rice bowls, and stuffed potatoes. Take the time to identify a few go-tos, and keep them in your freezer at home – work too, if there's space – so you never have an excuse to grab fast food.

- Many stores are offering big vats of soups and chili as well. These are often surprisingly good choices (check the nutrition information, as always), add a hard-boiled egg or piece of cheese if it's a little low in protein, and bypass the rolls or crackers on the side.

- Other go-to quick foods you'll find at the grocery store and might want to keep around include: individually wrapped cheddar or mozzarella sticks, string cheese, nut or seed butters (also available in single-serve packets if you lack refrigeration), fresh whole fruit, bags of washed and peeled carrots and celery, Greek yogurt or cups of coconut "yogurt," and healthy varieties of sliced organic deli style meat. Just from these things, you can throw together a very healthy meal. When I have "nothing" in the house, here's what I eat: half a package (3 1/2 ounces) of nitrate-free organic turkey, a cup of fresh fruit or seasonal berries, a handful of carrot sticks (or a big spoonful of whatever leftover cooked vegetables I have), and a yogurt or a couple of homemade gluten-free brownie bites. It's not glamorous, but it tastes good, keeps me going for a few hours, and satisfies my nutritional needs.

Learn how to adapt any restaurant meal or situation to meet your needs. One of the easiest ways to fail at your desired eating plan is by eating out too often, eating out at the wrong types of places, or making the wrong choices when you do eat out. It is definitely possible to be healthy when you eat out and, for the most part, you should continue to follow the guidelines above. A dietician can teach you more specifically how to do this, or there are many articles online describing a strategy for eating out at everything from ethnic restaurants to fast food chains. I believe that eating out – especially fine dining and multi-cultural dining – is one of life's pleasures. You just need to know how to handle it gracefully, so you can enjoy the food and company, without the follow-up feelings of disgust, self-loathing, and grossness that occur when you let yourself go hog-wild.

Learn how to cook. As mentioned above, you can fake it through the art of assemblage. However, it's just so much easier to learn the basics of cooking! Not only does it give you total control over the quality of your ingredients, you get everything made just the way you like it, and costs are dramatically less than eating out or buying even healthy prepared foods. If this is not one of your skills, you can learn some things from watching YouTube videos or the cooking channels, but there's nothing better than hands-on application of skills. If you have a friend or relative who is a good cook, get them to show you the basics. If not, look for cooking classes. There are private cooking classes offered by the gourmet cooking store chains, like Williams Sonoma or Sur La Table. Larger communities may have a private cooking school oriented toward laypeople, where you can take a four-class introduction to everything from fish to eggs to vegetables, meat, dessert, soups, salads and more. That's probably enough to get you going. There are also typically low-fee classes at your local adult school, taught on a nearby high school campus. Classes are also fun social occasions, especially if you take a friend. Then you can practice on each other.

Decrease anxiety about food and food-focused situations. I know, this is easier said than done. If you have a history of being overweight, or of engaging in eating disordered behavior, it can be really hard to go grocery shopping, let alone eat with other people. The fear of judgment is strong, as is the sense of shame. I'd like to be able to say you're imaging it, but the reality is that, despite more than a third of the general (non-PCOS) population being considered overweight or obese, people are incredibly judgmental about weight. Practice going from low-risk to higher-risk situations to increase your sense of comfort with just plain old eating. Start at home, or with a close friend. Take someone grocery shopping with you if that's an issue. Move on to the ultimate tests – stopping by a pastry or candy shop, for example. See what feelings come up and make note of them. It may be helpful to work some of that out in therapy. We've got enough to deal with, without being scared to simply eat.

Adopt a mindset of abundance, creativity, and accomplishment as it relates to your food. So many of us have restricted ourselves for so long, maybe even what feels like forever. I started my first diet when I was 10 years old, which was highly unusual for the time. Until a few years ago, I basically spent my entire life battling with food on some level. I know this is true for many of you as well. Shifting your mindset from restriction, limitation, and the idea of "good" and "bad" foods is important for your mental health and well-being, as well as the health of your body. Similarly, because of the way diets are taught to us, creativity is destroyed. Food becomes punishing, restrictive, and unpleasant. I would like you to start thinking about food as a potential source of fun and creativity, as well as abundance. Even if you have restrictions due to a true food allergy, celiac disease, or something else, you can find pleasure in food again. If you can start to shift your thinking, behavior will follow, and food will feel like a less pressured and punishing topic.

Allow yourself the occasional reasonable treat. The definition of reasonable can vary widely. I'm talking about considering your long-term goals against your short-term desires, and making choices that give you what you want, just not all the time, or in huge quantity. Treats should be personalized. I would be fine if I never had a mocha latte, but you might think you'd die if that was off your list of allowable foods forever. Good dark chocolate is a must have for me, while you might not even like chocolate. If someone told me my designated treat was a glass of wine, I would be really bummed out, even though I like wine. I'm happy with perhaps one cocktail per month, but you might like a few glasses of wine every week.

It has to be something that feels right for you, and you have to be honest about it. If I choose chocolate, that doesn't mean an entire three to four ounce European bar; it means one to two squares (about an ounce) of that bar. If it's wine, it's a small glass, not a giant goblet filled to the top or a bottle. You get the picture. I think these foods are important parts of our daily lives, memories, and culture. It would be sad to forever eliminate birthday cake or your grandma's old country ziti recipe. Unless you have an issue such as celiac disease or nut allergy, in which case you must always follow restrictions, the occasional treat will make you feel like you're not missing out on too much, but you're still doing the right thing for your body and your brain.

Changing Food Behaviors

Plan for every possible sabotage: restaurants, office birthdays, or dinner at grandma's house. Have you ever heard: "When you don't have a plan, you plan to fail?" So many women with PCOS report being "blindsided" by eating opportunities that caused them to go off track by making poor choices in the moment. Life is full of sabotage opportunities and things that will trigger cravings. Most of us are confronted with several every week, if not every day. It's the meals out, the snacks at the movies, the random candy dish, the church potluck, the television ad for your favorite burger place, or the cooking channel featuring your favorite red velvet cupcakes. I KNOW. I'm as subject to temptation as everyone. That is why you must have a plan.

- As much as possible, know where you're going ahead of time and what sort of food will (or won't) be available.

- If it's not easy to tell, call. This is part of becoming more assertive about your health. Call the conference center, the restaurant, or even your friend who is hosting dinner, so you can plan accordingly.

- If you're easily swayed by what your friends or family members are ordering, make a healthy choice before you even get to the restaurant, order first, and stick with it.

- Practice being assertive in challenging food situations. Head off trouble by offering two or three relatively healthy choices to others if you're going out with a group. Don't be afraid to take a sandwich from a luncheon buffet, pull the fillings out, and leave the bread on your plate. If you love your best friend's dinner parties, but all she serves is a giant salad and a bigger plate of pasta, take your own protein source, or eat it before you get there, so you don't feel unbalanced all evening. These are learned behaviors, and they will take time to master, but just start practicing.

- Going to grandma's house for Thanksgiving? This one is challenging. I don't think you should miss out on holidays, but again, planning strategically will leave you feeling better about yourself while still getting to enjoy things. It's better to have a few bites of the things you love the most, leave the stuff you don't care about, and not be set off on an eating binge and indulgence cycle that spans five or six weeks of the holidays.

Stop "dieting." Maybe you have heard: "Diet is a four-letter word." I agree. The fact is, 97% of people who go on a diet will regain the weight, and quite often, much more. PCOS is a lifetime disorder, and we have to think long-range. So, I like the term "eating plan" instead of the word diet. A diet is all about deprivation. An eating plan is something that can shift over time, as your needs change, and allows for flexible boundaries. That is a healthy approach!

Don't skip meals. There are many perspectives on when, how much, and how often you should eat for optimal health, weight loss, and good functioning: intermittent fasting, three squares a day, three meals and two to three snacks, or five to six mini meals. I have spent an inordinate amount of time considering this topic and trying out each of these formats. For the purposes of good brain health and functioning, I've come to the conclusion that simply eating three meals a day, with plenty of protein and not too many carbs, and without snacking (with the possible exception of a mid-afternoon snack if your dinner will be a little late), is the best approach. Your brain needs a steady supply of amino acids and glucose. But your PCOS body is highly likely to be insulin resistant, with a pancreas that's always struggling to stay on track. I buy off on the theory that giving your pancreas a break is a good idea. I also find that it's easier to get all the elements in a full meal: at least two vegetables and one fruit, along with healthy fat and protein, and some fun or tasty carbohydrates, like dark chocolate. When you're doing the mini meals approach, or multiple snacks, it's easier to justify going out of balance, get filled up on the wrong stuff, or skip actual meals in favor of just snacks, because snacks tend to be fun foods.

Get a *legitimate* nutritionist/dietician if you need more help. It can be really hard to implement these changes. Some information may be confusing, or conflict with something you've read or been told previously. So why do I put so much emphasis on *legitimate*? In my experience, credentials for medical doctors are pretty clear (you're either an MD or you're not), but credentials for nutritionists and dieticians are not nearly as clear. They also vary by location (certification, licensure, and registration may all be considered acceptable for practice). A registered dietician actually holds a clearly defined title, indicating the highest level of science-based training, education, and experience. A nutritionist does not; in fact, in many places, you can call yourself a nutritionist without any education or training in the field of nutrition! That's pretty scary because many medical diseases require very specifically calibrated nutritional plans.

Personal trainers, health coaches, nutrition coaches, or holistic health coaches can dispense nutritional information with as little as a five-day course in nutrition or a one-year certificate course. Many individuals, myself included, have a phenomenal amount of nutritional knowledge, but they are not registered dieticians, with all the specific training necessary to treat medical conditions. If you are very healthy and just want to lose a few pounds, an unlicensed nutritionist may offer useful advice. Otherwise, please start with someone whom you know is well trained, educated, and experienced in nutritional management – even better if that expertise includes PCOS.

Transitioning from Not so Healthy to Pretty Good to Great!

Keep a Food/Mood Log

It is critical to know your starting point, what the problem areas are, and what you want to achieve. Keeping a food/mood log for a full week is an excellent way to gather this information. What's included is typically: day/date/time you ate; what you ate and how much; whom you were with/where you were (for example, with your best friend, at a party, home on the couch); how you felt both before and after you ate (physically, mentally, and emotionally); why you ate (bored, angry, obligated etc.); other notes or reflections. Spending some time really analyzing this information can provide invaluable information about what you should focus on first. Here are the details of what you should be paying attention to in order to get the most out of this exercise:

Day/date/time you ate: for most people, there will be a significant variance in weekend versus weekday behavior. This will also reveal consistency or inconsistency in your eating habits, and potential trouble spots like skipping breakfast and then making a bad snack choice a few hours later. Many of us eat too late at night, just before bedtime, which can be a problem as well, especially for those of us with insulin resistance. Late night eating leads to increased weight, sleep problems, and acid reflux/gastroesophageal reflux disease (GERD).

What you ate and how much: Note what you ate, how it was prepared, and how much. Be very specific, and scrupulously honest. This information is only for you and will not be judged. Don't say "some fruit," but "three medium organic apricots." Instead of "some nuts," note "1/2 cup of salted and roasted mixed nuts." And not "a hamburger with all the fixings," but "a 1/3 pound burger from Jimmy's with one slice of cheese, three strips of bacon, fried onion pieces, a large white bun, ketchup, and two slices each of tomato and lettuce." It's really easy to hide the truth with vagueness. "I ate vegetables!" sounds pretty good, but when it's an entire deep-fried blooming onion from your favorite steakhouse, I call baloney! Nice try. Don't worry about trying to change your diet while you are doing this information gathering exercise, although you may notice some choices getting better, because your shame has been activated, or you are just more conscious.

Who you were with/where you were: For many people, it's easy to be "good" when they're in their weekday routine, but things fall apart when there's a special event (birthday parties, graduations, anniversary dinners), you're hanging out with certain people (spouse or lover, at your childhood home with all your relatives), or at certain times of day (at night, on the couch, after dinner) or settings (vacations, office parties, casinos, buffets). Many of these things may be emotional triggers, or it could simply be that you've gotten awfully relaxed and let your guard down. Or maybe you were drinking, and your decision-making got a little sloppy and all of a sudden, a giant pepperoni pizza appeared on your doorstep (it could happen!).

How you felt both before and after you ate (physically, mentally, and emotionally): Food really does affect mood. This is the most critical part of the exercise, because it provides motivation when you can see the direct effects of your eating behaviors on your mood, functioning, and sense of well-being. Sometimes you will eat (usually toward the healthier side of the spectrum), and you feel full, satisfied, clear-headed, energized, and ready to go. That's what we're aiming for. Other times, you feel like a slug, your brain is thick and heavy, you can't think clearly, and your motivation has been zapped (usually when you veer toward the unhealthier choices). When you eat things that are not good for YOUR body, your mood will be directly affected. Your body and your brain will crash, and you may get irritable, anxious, depressed, or unfocused. I don't think that's a good way to live.

Why you ate (bored, angry, obligated, etc.): This is also really critical information for getting a handle on your own personal eating demons. There's a helpful acronym, HALT: hungry, angry, lonely, or tired. When you're feeling any of those four things, and you eat, your eating is probably an attempt to self-medicate or self-soothe, not an attempt to simply fuel your body's energy needs. If you notice having a certain feeling is always followed by eating, that's an emotion that needs some attention. Sometimes obligatory eating, like your mom's food, or at a company meeting, or a birthday party, leads to poor choices as well.

Other notes or reflections: If you have diabetes and check your blood sugar daily, this would be recorded here. Similarly, if there are medications you take with meals, exercises you did, you got sick, you had your period, you were traveling (don't do this exercise when you're traveling, unless travel is part of your normal daily life, like you have a sales job), etc. would all go here. Also note any critical events that may affect mood, such as a death in the family, getting laid off, or getting injured.

Things You Can Do

Weigh yourself less often or not at all. Some people recommend throwing out the scale all together, and just using visual cues or the way your clothes fit as a guideline. That's perfectly fine. There's a really wide range of healthy or "acceptable" weights – the weights at which we feel relatively comfortable in our bodies. Some people weigh themselves once a day, once a week, or only at the doctor's office or gym. That's fine too. And some people weigh themselves multiple times a day, when they wake up, after they go to the bathroom, after they eat, and so on. Sorry, that's not fine; that's a symptom of an eating disorder.

So how often should you weigh yourself? Be reasonable about it. If you have a history of an eating disorder and know that the scale thing can get a little obsessive for you, then you need to limit it to once a week.

Maybe that means putting the scale in a really awkward place so it's not easy to grab multiple times a day, keeping it in someone else's bedroom, or something like that. Daily weigh-ins, along with blood sugar readings and sometimes blood pressure measurements, are part of my routine, but I don't panic if I can't weigh myself. My weight tends to fluctuate within about a five-pound range all the time, and I think that's fairly common for women with PCOS. I don't like that, but I accept it, and I appreciate the validation the scale gives when I'm feeling uncomfortable in my body.

Detox your diet. I don't mean go Hollywood and do a severely calorie-restricted liquid diet. I mean, start really looking at what's in your food and beverages, and start deleting the stuff that's really bad for you. Starting points: aspartame, artificial coloring, non-organic wheat, most sugars, juice, soda, commercially made smoothies, almost anything you can buy at a convenience store, anything you can't pronounce, anything with a disturbingly long expiration date on it (Twinkies are just plain scary, for example), nitrate and nitrites (commonly found in preserved meats, hot dogs, etc.), hydrogenated and partially hydrogenated fats (ubiquitous in crackers, chips, cookies, etc.), and fast food.

More simple guidelines: eat nothing with more than five ingredients, if you can't pronounce some of the ingredients, or if your grandmother would have no idea what this "food" is. And definitely listen to Michael Pollan (*The Omnivore's Dilemma*): "Eat food. Not too much. Mostly plants." Beyond that, it's all noise, and I suggest you ignore it.

Increase your dietary variety. This is actually kind of fun. Most people (some estimates are about 60% of us) eat the same two dozen or so foods over and over and over. This is due to cultivated preferences, ease, simplicity, and unwillingness to explore. I'm a firm believer in eating seasonally and eating as much variety as possible in general. I think there are innumerable trace minerals and other elements that come from foods that may only appear at certain times of year, or for a limited time. We may not know what those things are, but they're here for a reason, and I think they're part of good brain health. Buy all the weird looking fruits and vegetables at the farmers' market. Try the bison or the emu. I can't imagine that you wouldn't find a recipe on the internet. Go to a restaurant featuring cuisine from a place you've never heard of. It will be good for you. Aim to try one new food item or spice every time you buy groceries or eat out. The stuff that's relatively easy or tasty should get incorporated into your meal planning.

Stay positive. Question the messages you take in about weight, body, and food from society, friends, family, and especially the media. I could write an entire book on the topic of internalized negative messages, what that does to women's self-esteem, and how it alters behavior in undesirable ways. I'm not asking you to turn into a body positivity activist, but I am asking you to increase your consciousness, and be honest about what gets under your skin. If you are shamed about your size, attire, shape, or food preferences, it tends to incite alternating cycles of driven attempts at compliance and horrible outbursts of rebellion ("I'll show you what fat looks like!"). This form of "body rebellion" is usually unhealthy and the only one who really gets hurt is YOU.

Well-meaning relatives, teachers, coaches, friends, and doctors can say things that range from insensitive to downright cruel, especially when young women are entering puberty and their bodies are changing rapidly. You may have felt the punishing and judgmental eyes of people in line with you, pointedly checking out the size of your butt and the contents of your grocery basket. People at the office may ask "do you think you should be eating that?" as if it was actually their right to decide what's best for you. All of this is demoralizing, quietly enraging, and leads to a crushing loss of self-esteem. I want you to pay attention to who does this, when, and under what circumstances – and then start calling them out on it. Here's how to do it:

"I can't believe you just commented about the calorie content of what I ordered at the restaurant. It makes me really uncomfortable to know that you are monitoring my food, and I feel like you just don't trust me to make good choices. I want you to stop making comments like that immediately. I will feel so much better about our relationship when you respect my choices, and don't comment on them."

Fight media stereotypes. A lot of things are blamed on the media, sometimes rightly so. A media that favors ultra-skinny, unusually tall, mostly white, able-bodied, and exceptionally beautiful women has significantly facilitated the generally oppressive and judgmental depictions of women's bodies. This is unrepresentative of society as a whole. Of course, these beautiful people should be admired for their unique physical attributes – but so should we all! I enjoy fashion, style, and beauty, but I always dread seeing "the September issue" with 500+ pages of fashion layouts and a million full-color ads and seeing at best one or two images (not even pages, just images!) of women who don't fit the current beauty ideals. This is a constant assault on our senses (yes, "beauty" can be an assault on the senses!). Because again, it's something that infiltrates your brain, is held up as an ideal, and rewarded by almost everyone. Combat this by seeking out style, fashion, and beauty images (if you're in to such things) that are more congruent with reality: women with curves, petite women, dark skinned women, and women with unusual features. You will feel a little internal sigh of relief and affirmation, and that is one very important way in which we begin to combat that battered and bruised feeling that defines your self-esteem.

Grieve the habits you're giving up. Food is physical, emotional, intellectual, and cultural. Food is love for many of us, right? Food is powerful. Changing your lifelong eating habits is hard. I get it. I'm asking you to give up your favorites, the fast and easy stuff, and the stuff that tastes addictively good, for crying out loud! In the process, you are likely going to have to deal with some very real feelings of loss. I mean deep, real, profound grief, complete with some tears about giving up one thing and moving towards another. You are also going to have to deal with any other feelings that come about eating differently, feeling different, and quite possibly looking different as well. This is why I say to think of "one day at a time." You can adhere to a decision for a little while, without too much difficulty, but to think "I'm never going to be able to eat Uncle Carl's famous barbecue again" is a sure set-up for more rebellion, a binge, and possibly even a long drawn-out period of backsliding and woe while you look back at your accomplishments, slipping away rapidly, with misery.

Prepare to be noticed. As your body and behaviors begin to change, people will notice. And some of them won't like it and may even try harder to keep you stuck where you have been. They may feel threatened because you're getting more conventionally attractive, losing your identity as "the sick one," or eating stuff that looks unfamiliar or tastes different than what they're used to. You may be cooking less, or more, and that might be perceived as less fun. Certainly, your refusal of the white bread, the cheap tacos, or the double gulp cola may incite ire. People get funny that way. You would think that they're only interested in what they consume, but it isn't so, and you need to be prepared for it.

Prepare to feel better. You're also going to have to get real about your changing body and brain. Although one might assume that it's undesirable to feel sick, tired, foggy, lethargic, and gross, that can be hard to give up too. There's safety in the invisibility of being the fat chick, the sick one, or the depressed one. People might expect more of you when you're not somewhat incapacitated. You might expect more of yourself. You might have to start dating, or get sexual, or wear totally different clothes, or really own your life decisions. Those things can be scary, intimidating – even incapacitating. But that's a temporary thing, if you choose to work at it. You might need to go to therapy or do some other personal growth work to be able to fully step into the new you who believes in her future and her ability to manage her health and her body.

This chapter is a limited introduction to healthy diet as it relates to mental health and good brain functioning. I include it because I think diet is a critical part of mental health, and it's something I don't get to talk about nearly as much as I'd like to in private practice. This is an invitation to start exploring, bringing back foods you may have automatically banned for years, and seeing what feels right in YOUR body, not the imaginary body created by some diet book writer. I encourage you to start looking for solid resources about eating well; some of them are listed in the back of this book.

CHAPTER 10

Prescription Medications, Foods, and Procedures

O
ne of the most confusing things in the world of PCOS is prescription medications and supplements. Which ones should you take? Which ones are dangerous? Which ones are useless? Which ones only matter if you're trying to get pregnant? Research is limited, and doctors only have a limited range of approved options to offer. These medications often carry a high price as well, both financially and in terms of potential side effects. According to a 2015 report by IMS Institute for Healthcare Informatics, in 2014 Americans spent $375 BILLION on pharmaceuticals! Yet many of us have doubts about the intentions of "Big Pharma" and/or believe in the body's own natural healing abilities. Supplements are a $30 billion plus per year business in the United States. That's about $100 per person per year, if every single American was buying supplements. Since that's not the case, some of us are spending a whole lot more than $100/year. Not surprisingly, women with PCOS are a great potential audience for any cure for insulin resistance, quick weight reduction, or generally feeling better. It's a complex problem, and we are notorious for chasing every chance of a cure or at least relief.

The most commonly prescribed medications include birth control pills to regulate your cycle, metformin to improve insulin resistance, spironolactone for hair loss and hirsutism, and Clomid or Letrozole to help you conceive. For other medications, you will see a separate doctor for each bodily symptom or part. If you want natural cures, you will need to either find an alternative medicine practitioner or piece it together yourself through self-study. I am an advocate of both a very well-informed do-it-yourself approach, and of using the full complement of traditional and alternative healthcare providers as consultants and advisors.

Part of a therapist's responsibility is to monitor her client's medications, particularly psychotropic medications. Your therapist should ask about all your medications the first time you meet. It is your responsibility to report changes in medication to your therapist, although your therapist will likely ask for an update from time to time. I tend to take a very involved approach, including active coordination with the prescribing physician, because it leads to better patient care.

Because of the way medicine is typically administered, you are likely to have several physicians prescribing for you, and not necessarily communicating regularly with one another. Ideally, you would fill all your prescriptions at one pharmacy and have a personal relationship with the pharmacist, in order to have some oversight about potentially problematic interactions. Again, due to the realities of insurance and chain pharmacies, you're more likely to have a computerized medication interaction checker and a rotating team of pharmacists and pharmacy assistants who know very little about you or your condition. When you pick up your prescriptions, ask to speak to the pharmacist to find out about the likeliest potential side effects. If you have trouble remember the details, keep a list in your wallet or on your phone, so that you always know what you're taking.

I expect my clients to report medication changes to me as soon as they can, because sometimes side effects that look like psychological symptoms may develop (for example, depression developing or getting worse with birth control bills). I can't treat a condition that's being created by a medication, but I can provide guidance and refer you back to your doctor. By keeping your therapist in the loop about prescription medications and your other medical conditions, you're actually getting an extra set of eyes and ears. Because your therapist sees you week-to week, rather than daily, like your friends and family do, sometimes things are more noticeable to your therapist than the people you see daily. Your therapist can often help identify problems – or progress – that you might not see.

Never take medications without asking lots of questions. This seems obvious – we were all taught not to take pills if we didn't know what they were, where they came from, and what they're supposed to do. But over time, we may start to forget how important this is. Don't assume that what's prescribed is beneficial until you're sure you understand the potential benefits as well as side effects. Your doctor should have a clear, logical reason for prescribing a medication, and be able to explain it in terms you understand, along with possible side effects and alternatives. Sometimes you don't have a choice (say, when you're in the emergency room), but most of the time, you have time to do a little research. If you are questioning whether a medication is right for you, get on the internet, talk to your pharmacist, talk to friends or relatives who are medical professionals (or those who share the same condition), and see what else you can find out. If you have more questions, make a follow-up call or visit to your doctor.

Note that this is very different from saying "I don't want prescription medication, and I'm not doing it, so don't even talk to me about it." I think part of a balanced and self-loving approach to your health is to consider ALL the options. Ultimately, you may reject some or all of them, but at least listen, pause, consider, and then make your decision. You may not like the decision you feel you have to make, but at least you will understand it completely. Participating in and then owning a decision will feel a lot better than having a knee-jerk reaction to an idea you don't like. Sometimes the benefits can be amazing.

Case Example, Vanessa:

> Vanessa was a woman with PCOS who had been plagued with erratic periods, excessive bleeding, horrible cramping, and endometriosis. She'd had a couple of cysts surgically removed and it was strongly suspected that she also had fibroids. She was 42, still had vague thoughts of wanting children, and was advised to have

a hysterectomy. Vanessa was opposed to hysterectomy, because she'd heard that doctors over-prescribe it, and was worried that she would lose her sex drive. Finally, though, her symptoms became so bad, she relented and had the surgery. She experienced relief of all symptoms and got the bonus of no threat of uterine cancer. She regretted having suffered so much, just because she rejected an idea.

When you're feeling anxious or scared about a surgery or its potential complications, or wonder if it's truly necessary, it's hard to think clearly and really look at the big picture. Assessing risks using reliable statistics, consulting with trusted medical professionals (other than the potential surgeon), and taking a little time to consider the potential benefits in light of the potential for risks will help you make better decisions about your medical care, especially when it comes to "optional" surgeries.

Case Example, Candy:

Candy was a 25 year old woman with PCOS who had been dealing with irregular periods for over a decade. She also had terrible cramps and other PMS symptoms. She'd had a couple of pregnancy scares too. Her period – or lack thereof – was a constant problem. Her gynecologist recommended birth control pills, but Candy was into natural remedies and supplements. She thought birth control pills "messed with nature" and had to be bad. Besides, women could get blood clots and stuff! Her doctor encouraged her to do her own research. Candy was open-minded enough to do that, and spent some time doing additional research. She also spoke with two female relatives who had used birth control pills. Ultimately, she decided to try the pills. She started getting regular periods, her PMS symptoms were reduced, and she had a reliable form of birth control as a bonus. She felt really good about her decision, because she knew how the statistics applied to her specifically. What might be true for a 40 year old smoker wasn't true for her as an otherwise healthy 25 year old.

In Candy's case, although birth control pills weren't her first choice, she thought that the potential was there to receive a lot of benefit. She knew that if she tried them and didn't feel well, she could stop taking them without any problem. This made her feel comfortable enough to try them.

A Word of Caution

It's easy to get caught up in an anti-pharmaceutical/pro-natural mindset regarding prescription medication versus herbs and supplements. After all, we're talking about chemicals, record-breaking profits, and "Big Pharma" versus "pure, safe, organic, and natural." Like most things, the truth probably lies somewhere in the middle. The problems is, not knowing what's really true may be contributing to your stress level rather than enhancing your wellness!

Pharmaceuticals are tested, but we still don't know enough about most of them. Due to variable regulatory standards for supplements, and the potential for tremendous profit, supplements just may not be as reliable as you might think or hope. Before you make any decisions about pharmaceuticals or supplements, some of which I believe can definitely positively affect psychological conditions, it's important to understand more about how these things work. My focus is on psychotropic medications and other medications that may have psychological effects.

Psychotropic medications are powerful pharmaceutical compounds that may help control anxiety, depression, dysthymia, bipolar disorder, sleep disorders, schizophrenia, and a host of other conditions that present primarily in the mental health realm. They can range in their effects from miraculous, such an antidepressant lifting a person from a suicidal gloom, to ineffective (wrong drug, too low a dose), undesirable (weight gain, loss of libido), or fatal (deliberate overdoses, seizures caused by abrupt withdrawal, or Stevens Johnson syndrome, a very rare reaction to certain drugs that starts with a rash). I wish it was a "one pill cures all" sort of thing, but it's not.

Medications commonly prescribed to women with PCOS include metformin, spironolactone, birth control pills, antidepressants, mood stabilizers, antipsychotics, sleep aids, appetite suppressants, and anxiolytic medications. In addition to the pills we think of as medication, there are some other things that may be prescribed for mental health disorders. These are classified as medical foods, prescription supplements, and medical procedures. They include Deplin, customized Chinese herbal formulations, ketamine syrup, transcranial magnetic stimulation (TMS), and electro-convulsive therapy (ECT). I include them because, in treating long-term depression, sometimes you need to look beyond the obvious. I'm also including some things, like metformin, that aren't necessarily mental health treatments, but may have mental health side effects, because it's important to know what's causing (or helping) what. Additionally, I'll take a brief look at medical marijuana or its components (THC and CBD), ketamine, TMS, and ECT.

The Prescribing Process

You may have heard the term "off-label uses" in reference to prescription medication, and wonder if there's some hopeful news for you in there. The answer, like so many things in medicine, is a qualified "maybe." First of all, what does the term actually mean? In the United States, it means that the Federal Drug Administration (FDA) has approved a medication to treat a certain disease or symptom. The approval process is complex and expensive. Manufacturers usually choose to study, test, and submit documentation for the most potentially profitable aspect. But there are other uses that may be perfectly safe, legal, appropriate, and helpful. It's just that the FDA hasn't specifically approved them for that use. Examples of this include:

- Trazodone, an antidepressant, is often prescribed for sleep (and also appetite control).
- Lamictal for bipolar disorder and seizures may also be prescribed for impulsive behavior or mood swings.
- Wellbutrin for stopping smoking is often prescribed as a primary antidepressant, and for PMS symptoms.
- Cymbalta, an antidepressant, is also used to treat anxiety, neuropathy, fibromyalgia, and chronic pain.

It sometimes seems rather hasty the way doctors can dispense a prescription or two or three so quickly. This may leave you wondering if the prescribed medication is actually the best choice for you. Choosing a medication may seem like a quick decision to your physician, but he or she has prescribed a lot of medication for the same or similar conditions. However, just because it takes two seconds to scribble a prescription doesn't mean it isn't a well-considered medical opinion and option coming at you from that prescription pad. Some diseases are easier to treat than others, but a lot of the ones that affect women with PCOS require some trial and error. Thyroid levels need to be quite precise, for example, and there are several classes of medications for both diabetes and high blood pressure. What works well for one person may cause unpleasant side effects for another, or not work at all. Be patient with the process, ask plenty of questions, and be sure to report both positive and negative symptoms or experiences while taking medication. It's also possible to feel absolutely no change at all, and this should be reported to your doctor as well.

When it comes to psychotropic medications, the process can be even more complex. Unfortunately, although there are some developments in neurotransmitter testing which may eventually point the way toward the most effective medications for a particular patient, these tests are not commonly used yet. That means the process remains more of an educated guess. The history of your own medication trials as well as family history can be helpful. If you've previously used a medication and found it to be effective, you may simply be able to re-start that medication. Or, if you have never been on medication, but you have a family member who has been on medication that works well for their depression, anxiety, etc., that's often a good starting point, as a medication that worked well for your sister is likely to be one of your best choices as well.

One thing I would like to emphasize is that going to a therapist does NOT mean you will be automatically referred to a psychiatrist for a medication evaluation. Quite the contrary, unless you are in a crisis (feeling suicidal, or unable to go to work because of your symptoms). For mild and moderate mood disorders, talk therapy is just as effective, if not more so, than prescribed medication. For severe disorders (particularly bipolar disorder and schizophrenia, both of which almost always require medication), that is less true. But if, in my professional assessment, I think you will benefit from talk therapy, and you don't want to consider medication, I don't have a problem with that if you are not in danger. In fact, I respect your motivation and your desire to get through this thing on your own, by learning better skills and processing your feelings and experiences. But if things don't improve over time, I may raise the issue again. Just know that it's not a gratuitous suggestion. It's also not an order; it's something I'm going to want to discuss thoroughly.

I've seen many patients who are vehemently anti-medication, which often comes because of mistrust of the psychiatric system. They may have seen someone else suffer from serious side effects, particularly in the early days of psychotropic medications, when there was a stronger, yet less precise, group of medications. Or they may have tried a medication or two, gained weight or lost libido, and said "forget it!" You should definitely raise these concerns with your therapist, so that you can discuss them. Your therapist should be able to help you find someone who is a good personality match for you, and an expert in your type of condition. Your therapist should also ask you to sign a release form that allows the therapist to speak with the psychiatrist. When the treating therapist and psychiatrist are in regular communication with one another, it can be really helpful. They can combine their expertise, observations, and recommendations so that you get the best possible treatment. A strong partnership like this can be protective for you, and can also help you manage your medication options more quickly and effectively.

There are some other important things to know about psychotropic medications. The guiding principle is generally to prescribe the least possible dose that will give the most benefit, but there are definitely standardized doses. Sometimes, however, therapeutic effect is achieved with a lower than expected dose. People are more or less sensitive to the effects of prescription medications depending upon things such as age, gender, and weight. So, it's possible that a woman will require a different dose than a man, or perhaps a lower dose after losing weight.

Also, sometimes you need a combination of medications to achieve optimal symptom relief. That is why I recommend seeing a psychiatrist right from the start, or particularly if the first medication you try with your internist or general practitioner doesn't work well. A "cocktail" of medications that work on different neurotransmitters, or different classes of medications, may work better for you. In some cases, I've seen clients who took as many as four medications, each at a low dose, in order to reach optimal functioning.

Sometimes you need a long-term maintenance medication coupled with access to fast-acting or occasional use medications. An example would be an anti-anxiety medication or antidepressant that you take every day, but also having a prescription for a fast-acting anxiety medication for times when you experience intense anxiety. Anti-depressants will often help with sleep, but you may also be given a prescription for a sleep medication, like Ambien or Lunesta.

Antidepressants

In addition to treating depression, anti-depressants may also be prescribed for help with managing anxiety, insomnia, eating disorders, social anxiety, panic disorder, dysthymia (mild chronic depression, which frequently affects women with PCOS), ADHD, and pain management. That is why a doctor sometimes suggests an antidepressant, even if you don't report feeling depressed.

Here are general categories of antidepressants, along with some of their generic names, the neurotransmitters they act on, and the brand names of some of the more popular ones:

Selective Serotonin Reuptake Inhibitors (SSRIs): SSRIs are one of the most commonly prescribed antidepressants. They tend to have less side effects than earlier versions of antidepressants, although many of the older drugs are still useful. They've also been found to be useful for anxiety, some eating disorders, insomnia, and pain control. SSRIs help by blocking the reabsorption (reuptake) of serotonin in certain cells in your brain, leaving more serotonin available and improving mood. Some names of SSRIs are citalopram (Celexa), escitalopram (Lexapro), fluoxetine (Prozac), fluvoxamine, paroxetine (Paxil), sertraline (Zoloft), and vilazodone (Viibryd).

Side effects may include insomnia, sleepiness, weight gain, and loss of libido. SSRIs typically start to have some effect around three weeks and take about six weeks to reach full effectiveness. Unfortunately, they don't work for everyone. That means they may help you, and they may not – or they may help, but not enough. If one SSRI doesn't work for you though, don't give up. Another medication in the SSRI category might work, or you can try other categories of medications.

Serotonin and norepinephrine reuptake inhibitors (SNRIs): Like SSRIs, SNRIs work by inhibiting reabsorption of neurotransmitters, in this case serotonin and norepinephrine. They are considered to be highly effective for anxiety as well. Common names include duloxetine (Cymbalta), venlafaxine (Effexor), and desvenlafaxine (Pristiq). Side effects may include insomnia, headaches, sexual dysfunction, upset stomach, and minor increases in blood pressure.

In addition to the SSRIs and SNRIs, which are the most popular categories of antidepressants due to their more tolerable side effects, there are many older classes of medications that may be useful too. One benefit is that these medications are almost all available as generics now, which makes them more cost-effective. These medication classes include:

Selective Norepinephrine reuptake inhibitors (N-RIs): These medications block the action of the norepinephrine transmitters, and act as a reuptake inhibitor for norepinephrine and epinephrine (adrenaline). Reboxetine is a common prescription name. These drugs are typically stimulating and may also be useful for neuropathic pain and anxiety disorders. Dry mouth and nausea are common side effects.

Norepinephrine dopamine reuptake inhibitors (NDRIs): The most well-known of these is bupropion (Wellbutrin), which is one of my favorite medications due to the fact that it doesn't result in weight gain and doesn't reduce libido. Wellbutrin is also prescribed as an aid to stop smoking and can be helpful in regulating the mood swings associated with bipolar disorder. Dry mouth, nausea, and stomach pain are the most common side effects.

Tricyclic antidepressants (TCAs): These include amitriptyline, nortriptyline, clomipramine, dothiepin, doxepin, imipramine, and trimipramine. They increase norepinephrine and serotonin and block the action of acetylcholine, another neurotransmitter. It is believed that this combination rebalances the brain. Side effects include sedation, blurred vision, constipation, and dry mouth.

Reversible inhibitors of monoamine oxidase (RIMAs): Moclobemide is the common name for this medication. The RIMAs work by reducing the activity of monoamine oxidase, which breaks down into serotonin and noradrenaline. Side effects include sleep disturbance, agitation, dizziness, sleepiness, and dry mouth.

Tetracyclic/noradrenergic antidepressants (TCAs) such as mianserin and amitriptyline were introduced in the 1970s. They are considered to be first-generation antidepressants. People with low blood pressure or heart problems should not take these medications. The side effects are more severe and include trouble breathing, hives, agitation, restlessness, dry mouth, fast heartbeat, etc. However, because of the strong drying effect, TCAs are effective at very low doses to help improve diarrhea-predominant IBS, which affects many women with PCOS. The dose is typically not enough to provide an antidepressant effect.

Tetracyclic analogues of mianserin (sometimes called noradrenergic and specific serotonergic antidepressant or NaSSA), such as mirtazapine or Tolvon, are called atypical antidepressants. They have a bigger list of side effects, like dry mouth, constipation, and drowsiness, as well as some potential for problems if you abruptly stop the medication.

MAOIs (monoamine oxidase inhibitors), such as phenelzine (Nardil) and tranylcypromine were the first class of antidepressants ever developed. They interact with numerous drugs and foods, which can be problematic, as patients must eliminate those foods that contain tyrosine, such as aged cheeses, certain meats and fish, fermented (alcohol) beverages, and even some overripe fruits like bananas and avocados.

Melatonergic antidepressants such as agomelatine are much newer, and they are better in terms of unwanted sleep side effects, leaving patients without a "sleep hangover" in the morning.

Mood stabilizers may be prescribed for bipolar depression, as well as for dysthymia and major depressive disorder. These include Lamictal, lithium, Tegretol, and Depakote. Side effects may include nausea, vomiting, diarrhea, trembling, weight gain, and drowsiness.

Anti-psychotic and atypical anti-psychotic (newer versions) **medications** may also be used to treat depression and bipolar disorder. Some of the more common ones include Clozaril, Latuda, Zyprexa, Seroquel, and Risperdal. Many patients find that adding an anti-psychotic medication to an antidepressant gives them a better overall result. Side effects include blurred vision, dry mouth, drowsiness, and weight gain.

Anti-Anxiety Medications

Medications to help you deal with anxiety may be fast-acting, short-term medications, or longer and slower-acting medications. Popular anti-anxiety medications may include the anti-depressants listed above, particularly the SSRIs, SNRIs, and tricyclics. Benzodiazepines (tranquilizers) and ketamine (as a syrup or infusion) are also prescribed for anxiety. Benzodiazepines are used for short-term management of anxiety. They include alprazolam, clonazepam (Klonopin), diazepam, and lorazepam (Xanax). They tend to produce almost immediate anxiety reduction, as well as muscular relaxation. However, long-term use may cause increased tolerance and the need for ever-higher doses, which may result in addiction. Benzodiazepines are therefore NOT a good long-term treatment for anxiety. Tricyclic antidepressants such as amitriptyline, imipramine, and nortriptyline may be helpful for anxiety, but can cause problems with blood pressure, constipation, dry mouth, blurry vision, and urinary retention. Ketamine (see below) may also be used for anxiety.

Medications for Sleep

If you have tried behavioral changes like adhering to a set sleep schedule, exercising, lowering stress, limiting caffeine, and eliminating daytime naps, yet still suffer from insomnia, you may need prescription sleep medication. Insomnia, by the way, can mean having trouble falling asleep, staying asleep, or waking too early to get adequate rest. These medications may also help if you suffer from intermittent insomnia due to a work or travel schedule that disrupts your routine, or in periods of acute stress. Prescription sleeping pills are either benzodiazepines, which depress the central nervous system, or antidepressants with a sedating effect. Before considering medication, read *Chapter 5* on sleep, and implement as many recommendations as you need.

Some antidepressants can be sedating when used at lower doses or an antidepressant may have the dual effect of improving depression and decreasing insomnia. Some of these include amitriptyline, Remeron, and trazodone. Trazodone is considered non-addictive and very safe, so it is one of the better choices. Common benzodiazepine generic and brand names include doxepin, estrazolam, Lunesta, Rozerem, Restoril, Halcion, Sonata, Ambien, and extended release Ambien CR.

Side effects of sleeping pills are many and varied, and can include feeling groggy upon waking, lightheadedness, dizziness, headache, a "sleep hangover," diarrhea, nausea, allergic reactions, sleep-eating, sleep-driving, sleep-walking, dry mouth, and problems with memory and performance of daytime activities.

Additionally, sleeping pills are not considered safe for many people. You should avoid alcohol when taking sleeping pills and be careful about starting or stopping them. There may be rebound insomnia when you go off them. They should almost always be used as a last resort, not a first choice, and underlying medical problems or health issues should be treated first.

Other Prescription Treatment Options

Proprietary/Custom-Blended Chinese Herbal Formulations. As with western medicine, Chinese herbs come in both prescription and over-the-counter versions. The latter are referred to as "patent medicine" and follow centuries-old formulations for specific conditions. If you see an acupuncturist or practitioner of Traditional Chinese Medicine (TCM), they may prescribe or prepare a customized herbal formulation to support the work they do with needles, massage, dietary recommendations, and other behavioral changes. These medications may be compounded in creams, gels, ointments, serums, powders, tonics, or capsules. TCM treats the entire body as a system, but there are specific treatments for anxiety and depression, as well as herbs that support good mental health.

While the herbs may be available without a prescription, they are indeed medications, and should be treated as such. Side effects are much less likely than with typical western prescription medications, but they do happen. Be sure to ask your practitioner what to expect, and when and what, if any, side effects may be expected. Some herbs can interact with drugs or may be unsafe for people with certain medical conditions. Some herbs are strong enough to cause miscarriage.

Medical Marijuana (Cannabis). As of 2017, over half of America's states, plus the District of Columbia, have legalized marijuana for either medicinal or recreational use, or both. For many other countries, this is increasingly true as well. Due to conflicting legal status (for example, legal in California, not legal at the Federal level), there has been somewhat limited research, but this is changing rapidly. Current research is focusing on potentially beneficial treatments for arthritis, alcoholism, diabetes, chronic pain, depression, and PTSD, among other conditions. Cannabis is a plant that contains cannabinoids, which act on the body's endocannabinoid (ECB) system. For medical purposes, the active parts of interest are tetrahydrocannabinol (THC) and Cannabidiol (CBD). THC is the part that gives you the euphoric feelings, or "high." CBD, which comprises about 40% of the plant's extract, is a cannabis compound that doesn't make you feel "stoned," counteracts the psychoactive effects of the THC, and has significant medicinal benefits. These benefits appear to include reducing inflammation, helping with nausea, decreasing pain, improving anxiety, and decreasing seizures. CBD also has neuro-protective benefits. In order to purchase medical marijuana, you typically need a medical marijuana card issued by a medical doctor, so that you can visit a dispensary (basically, a marijuana pharmacy) to fill your prescription.

Medical marijuana can be smoked, vaped, taken in an oil or tincture, applied topically, or eaten. Ratios of THC to CBD typically range from 1:1 to 1:18. It is difficult to find specific recommendations for dosing, but high ratios of CBD to THC appear to be the most effective for medical purposes. As with anything, starting at the lowest dose, and with caution, is recommended. What about the well-known side effect of marijuana causing "the munchies?" Apparently, this is not an issue with CBD-rich products. I am very curious to see how the research evolves, as the potential of medical marijuana for reducing inflammation and even insulin resistance is promising.

Ketamine (street name "Special K") is categorized as a "dissociative anesthetic," meaning it causes you to experience a detached, dreamlike state. It is a powerful drug. Ketamine is primarily an animal sedative, but it is now being used more extensively in human beings. Ketamine is fast-acting, but also wears off quickly – typically in no more than a week to 10 days. The side effects, such as depression, delirium, and impaired motor function, can last for 24 hours. It is abused for its hallucinogenic qualities. It is mainly used for starting and maintaining anesthesia and for pain management. There are now ketamine clinics that claim to treat mood disorders (even treatment resistant depression) and chronic pain, including migraines and nerve pain, with infusions of ketamine.

It has been shown to be rapidly effective for managing suicidal depression and intense anxiety. It may also have neuro-protective and anti-inflammatory effects. Ketamine may be provided as an injection in the emergency room. Emergency doses work in minutes, instead of days or weeks. The antidepressant effects of a single dose of ketamine may last for a week or longer. It is available in topical form and as a compounded syrup for pain, but also comes as a powder which may be snorted. It is sometimes used in conjunction with electroconvulsive therapy. Short and long-term side effects may include alterations in blood pressure and heart rate, nausea, vomiting, numbness, depression, hallucinations and cravings for the drug. One of the biggest problems with ketamine is that it does get you "high," which results in potential addiction problems. I have had patients who have used it with some success orally, topically, and as an injection in conjunction with electro-convulsive therapy, which is further described below. It is illegal to abuse ketamine, which is a controlled substance, but it is legal when appropriately prescribed and used.

Trans Cranial Magnetic Stimulation (TMS) is a non-invasive procedure in which nerve cells in the brain are stimulated by magnetic fields. It may improve depression, anxiety, obsessive compulsive disorder and other psychological conditions. It is not considered a first-choice treatment, but rather a choice when other treatments haven't been effective. The procedure involves placing an electromagnetic coil against your scalp while you sit in a chair in a medical clinic. The electromagnet delivers an external magnetic pulse to your brain in targeted areas that affect mood and depression. It is not entirely clear how it works, but the success rate is reported at about 30%, about the same as antidepressants at 14 weeks. TMS seems to work better on people who haven't "failed" a lot of antidepressants. The treatment is considered safe, but the patient may experience mild side effects such as headache, lightheadedness, tingling scalp and twitching or spasms of the facial muscles. More severe side effects could include seizures or mania. It is an expensive procedure that is not universally covered by insurance.

Electroconvulsive Therapy (ECT) is a procedure that is performed under general anesthetic. It has been used since at least the late 1930s. During that time, it has become a very refined and specific procedure. It has been incorrectly called "shock therapy" for decades, which has contributed to a continued fear of a procedure that is 70% to 90% effective for long-term, treatment-resistant depression. It works relatively rapidly on suicidal or catatonic patients. If you have "tried everything" for your depression, I am likely to refer you to an ECT expert for consultation about the possibility of using it for your treatment.

ECT may be administered as an inpatient or outpatient procedure.

Typically, it is administered two to three times a week for a total of six to 12 sessions, but may be administered daily for severe depression. If you are receiving ECT, you will be given a muscle relaxant and anesthetic. Electrodes are applied to the scalp and small amounts of electrical current are passed through the brain, which triggers a controlled seizure. Beyond that, it's still unclear exactly how ECT produces its often "miraculous" benefits. Side effects may include short-term memory impairment that gets better over time, nausea, headache, jaw pain, or muscle ache. Occasional follow-up sessions (every few months) may be necessary to maintain benefit, but many people never need another treatment.

Other Medications That May Have Psychological Effects

Diabetes Medications: Metformin, the most common prescription medication for insulin resistance or type 2 diabetes, doesn't seem like a medication that you would think has psychological side effects. And yet, because it tends to deplete Vitamin B12 over time, it can contribute to impaired cognitive (brain) function, some of that "brain fog" we're always talking about. Fortunately, supplementation with Vitamin B12 is cheap, easy, and effective. There is more information about Vitamin B12 in *Chapter 11.*

Gastrointestinal Medications: Excess abdominal weight may cause or contribute to gastrointestinal (GI) problems, including acid reflux. Many women with PCOS have a history of an eating disorder. If you have forced yourself to vomit (purge) or overeaten consistently to such a point that you involuntarily vomit, such as in Bulimia or Binge Eating Disorder, this may be another factor contributing to GI problems. The body is designed to tolerate occasional vomiting but doesn't do so well with frequent purging. This is not just an inconvenient or uncomfortable thing. Long-term untreated Gastroesophageal Reflux Disease (GERD) or heartburn can lead to esophageal erosion, which may set you up for esophageal cancer. Don't just pop an over-the-counter antacid and assume everything is fine. If you are experiencing a lot of heartburn, it's important to see a gastroenterologist for GERD assessment and possible prescription medications to stave off long-term irreversible damage. Long-term severe heartburn may also be an indicator of heart disease.

Additionally, because so many women with PCOS have diabetes (up to 50% of us) or pre-diabetes, it's important to know that diabetes leads to slow stomach emptying, which means that acid is prone to lingering longer than it should, resulting in reflux. Dietary changes are often the first step to managing reflux/GERD. Usually, you will be asked to limit fat, alcohol, tomatoes, chocolate, vinegar, citrus, and a number of other foods. These sorts of elimination diets are difficult for most patients to follow, even when they provide significant relief. The problem is, depending upon your specific symptoms, you may end up on yet another cocktail of medications prescribed by a gastroenterologist, perhaps as many as five if you have severe problems. Some of those medications may cause long-term side effects such as osteoporosis. It's important to treat the causes – excess weight, diet, and stress – not just the symptoms. If you must take prescription medications such as proton pump inhibitors (PPIs) to manage GI problems, limit the time and quantity as much as possible. The PPIs have a long list of associated side effects.

Elsewhere, we've talked a little about the gut/brain connection. Most of your serotonin (a "feel good" neurotransmitter) is produced in the gut. There is increasing evidence that women with PCOS suffer from an unbalanced gut microbiome, which may contribute to insulin resistance as well as depression. If your gut is off, it stands to reason that your serotonin is affected. Additionally, long-term antacid use may suppress your gut so that folate becomes depleted. Psychological effects of diminished folate include depression and irritability. Iron may also become depleted, which can contribute to chronic fatigue, hair loss, and anxiety. Vitamin B12 deficiencies may also occur, with resulting confusion, depression, and even dementia-like symptoms. Magnesium may become depleted with long-term use of these medications as well, which contributes to depression. Finally, Vitamin D may not be sufficiently "activated" if you're on these medications, again affecting mood/depression. These medications are very effective and sometimes necessary to prevent further damage to your body, but they should be considered in the context of their potential for psychological side effects as well.

Blood Pressure Medications: There are many different types of medications designed to lower high blood pressure. Some have a tendency to produce psychological side effects, and others do not. One such class is beta blockers, which make your heart beat more slowly, and with less force. This may reduce anxiety. Beta blockers, however, also contribute to depression and insomnia.

High Cholesterol Medications: Women with PCOS often have high cholesterol and dietary changes are usually the first recommendation to get it under control. If that doesn't work, your doctor will most likely prescribe a Statin to lower your cholesterol. The goal is reduction of heart disease risk, since women with PCOS are more prone to cardiovascular disease. Statin drugs can be very powerful, and side effects may include headaches, unpleasant nerve sensations, pain, bloating and diarrhea. On the psychological side, side effects may include noticeable memory impairment. Since this is also a common symptom of hypothyroidism and may be part of the overall fatigue and brain fog experienced by PCOS patients, it can be difficult to sort out the cause of your symptoms. It might seem like getting your cholesterol numbers as low as possible is good, but that's not necessarily true. Only your doctor can tell you what appropriate cholesterol levels are for you with your unique mix of conditions but do know that it actually IS possible for cholesterol levels to go too low, thereby causing or contributing to anxiety or depression. If you notice new symptoms or worse symptoms after starting a Statin, report the side effects to your doctor.

Thyroid Medications: The other common medications prescribed to women with PCOS are medications for **hypo**thyroidism, since again, so many of us are hypothyroid (the opposite condition, **hyper**thyroidism, is much less common). The thyroid controls metabolism, growth, muscle strength, appetite, body temperature, and reproduction, among other things. Hypothyroid symptoms include fatigue, weight gain, dry hair, brittle hair, cold intolerance, memory problems, depression, irritability, high cholesterol, and sluggish bowel. Because it is key to the functioning of every system in your body, it is critical to treat hypothyroidism correctly. Synthroid, typically prescribed as brand name only, is the synthetic thyroid that most doctors prescribe. Some doctors prescribe natural forms of thyroid, such as Armour Thyroid. Getting your thyroid corrected can "fix" innumerable symptoms and may even cause a little weight loss. Women represent 80% of all hypothyroid patients and it is important to test for thyroid conditions regularly when you have PCOS, because the picture can change over time. Significant dietary changes or other illnesses may change your dosing requirements. If you are taking too much thyroid medication for your hypothyroidism, you could end up with symptoms of anxiety. This happens sometimes when you are first starting on medication or changing doses of medication. Don't assume that this is just how it's going to be; describe your symptoms to your doctor so that appropriate adjustments can be made to alleviate these symptoms.

Allergy and Asthma medications: The first thing to know is that allergies are a big deal! Being symptomatic most of the time or all of the time can be exhausting, as your body is constantly fending off "invaders." The sneezing, itching, rashes, irritated eyes and nose can all contribute to poor mood and increased depressive symptoms. While it's not believed that allergies cause depression, it is known that they can contribute to it, and that people who have allergies are more likely to have depression. Some antihistamines, which are used to treat allergies, may also contribute to depression. Women with allergies have more asthma, and women with PCOS have – you guessed it – more of both. The steroids or corticosteroids prescribed to asthma patients and for topical allergies can contribute to a feeling of being sped up, anxious, or irritable. Additionally, steroids may cause significant rapid weight gain.

Conclusion

I hope all this information doesn't make you want to swear off prescription medications forever. I truly believe that there can be a place for them within a balanced and intelligent health-care plan. Sometimes they save lives, and sometimes they just make life more tolerable, or stave off negative long-term effects. The list of possible prescription medications and treatments is huge. If you need some assistance, don't be ashamed, and please don't give up after trying only one or two medications. There are many possible medications, combinations of medications, dosages, and ways of compensating for side effects. And, of course, there are also many natural, alternative remedies, herbs, and supplements, and procedures which are addressed more fully in the next chapter on supplements.

CHAPTER 11
Selective Supplementation and Other Tools

Prescription psychotropic medications are not always effective, may have strong side effects, may be costly for patients, or a patient may simply prefer to try a natural approach first. Supplements, herbs, and homeopathic remedies also have varying degrees of effectiveness, some side effects, or significant costs associated with them. Never assume that just because you can buy it without a prescription, it's automatically safe.

Always consult with your MD before starting any new supplements. Some supplements may interfere with prescription medications or cause other adverse effects.

While typical antidepressant medications alter reuptake (the reabsorption of a neurotransmitter by a neurotransmitter transporter after it has performed its function) or prevent breakdown of neurotransmitters, the supplements that interest me are the building blocks of the neurotransmitters. Ultimately, a carefully customized assortment of prescription medications, supplements, herbs, or homeopathic remedies will probably be the best approach. I have used herbs, homeopathic remedies, and supplements from traditional Chinese medicine (TCM), Ayurveda (traditional Indian medicine), allopathic (western) medicine, and traditional European homeopathy, as well as contemporary formulas from a variety of manufacturers.

Supplements and homeopathic remedies are commonly used in Europe and other countries to treat depression. Up to 64% of women with PCOS have depression. Many have anxiety, sleep issues, or other mood disorder issues. In addition to all the supplements that may be useful for PCOS, there are a number of supplements that may be helpful specifically in regulating mood. Note that, while sleep disorders are a distinct category of diagnosis, they can be treated by some of the same supplements, and across categories (they are also addressed in the prior chapter on prescription medications).

This chapter addresses a selection of relevant supplements, including herbs, along with some non-pharmaceutical treatments such as light therapy. Supplements, quite simply, are substances designed to provide nutrition that we may not get from other sources. There are literally thousands of supplements available over the counter. Some of them are single item (Vitamin C, Vitamin B12), some are combination products designed to maximize both components (glucosamine/chondroitin), and some are proprietary blends (a women's multi-vitamin, a doctor's house brand of "gut formula"). They are available almost everywhere. They range widely in price, effectiveness, and quality. And, they're a little bit controversial. Some people swear by them and others say all they do is give you the world's most expensive urine. I say you have to decide for yourself, and here are my thoughts on many of them that are relevant to mental health.

Most women with PCOS seem to be interested in trying supplements. Over the years, I have experimented with dozens, if not hundreds, of supplements. Currently, I use several supplements on a regular basis, including Vitamin D3, Vitamin C, N-Acetyl Cysteine (NAC), turmeric, lithium orotate, cinnamon, and berberine. I'll explain the "why" of my personal choices as I talk in more detail about each of these, as well as many others. **Always consult a medical professional who is familiar with the specifics of your body, prior history, family history, and health goals before adding or changing supplements.**

Just as I need to know about any prescription medications you're taking, I would definitely want to know what kind of supplements you're taking, why you're taking them, and what kind of results you've observed (if any) from your supplements. I ask these questions to screen for some possible problems, determine your willingness and ability to experiment with your treatment, and determine how you might benefit from strategic supplementation. I might also discuss whether you even want to pursue supplements as part of your health plan. But why would I consider offering such a contrary point of view, when we all know women with PCOS need lots of supplements? Here's why:

- Some supplements may require monitoring. Examples include Vitamin D levels, DHEA/Pregnenolone, and lithium orotate. Depending upon your basic level of health, other medications or supplements being consumed, as well as other factors, what's safe and effective for one person could be useless or counterproductive in another.

- You can overdose on them – rarely, but it's possible! I used to work with a woman who was taking so much Vitamin A, which is commonly found in carrots, because she thought it was good for her eyes, that her skin actually turned yellowish-orange!

- Sometimes they interact with other medications or herbs or supplements, and some of those other things may be a higher priority.

- All healthcare providers are not equally knowledgeable about the effects or interactions of supplements.

- Some supplements, like St. John's Wort, may need to be discontinued temporarily prior to surgery, or immediately after surgery.

- Sometimes they work the opposite of the way they're expected to work (for example, a small percentage of people who try 5-HTP to help them sleep will find that it has the effect of making their insomnia worse).

- Supplements can produce detrimental side effects (such as diarrhea from too much magnesium, which is a laxative in large doses).

- Sometimes they don't work at all, and you've just wasted money dumping useless stuff into your body.

- They're not covered by insurance.

- Some supplements may be challenging to source and difficult to compare (even with internet resources).

- It's easy to forget to take them at appropriate times. Some of the more complex programs of supplementation may require you take supplements up to six or eight times per day, carefully timed and spaced before, after, or with food. I don't know about you, but for most of us, we're doing well if we manage to take a few in the morning and a few more in the evening. This can be overwhelming and cause you to give up on supplements altogether.

- It's hard to differentiate what you're deriving benefit from, or how much useful substance you're getting. If you're also using your best source – your diet – the total intake is incalculable. If you're at all prone to obsessive tracking, it can take way too much time.

All this being said, I'm a believer in targeted supplementation, for limited periods of time. There's so much we simply don't know about nutrition and the micro-nutrients that are found in our foods. We may be eating foods from contaminated or depleted sources, too much processed food that has been stripped of nutrients, or have other stressors or health conditions that cause deficiencies. A deficiency of any of the following can be associated with various degrees of mental disturbance: Vitamin B1, Vitamin B3, Vitamin B6, Biotin, Folic acid, Vitamin B12, Vitamin D, Vitamin E, Calcium, Magnesium, Potassium, Zinc, Copper, Iron, essential fatty acids (EPA, DHA, GLA), and amino acids. In other words, if anything's missing, or over-represented, or under-represented, you may end up functioning sub-optimally.

Some of the symptoms of deficiency include depression, insomnia, irritability, mental confusion, dementia, delirium, lethargy, sleep disturbances, PMS, neurological problems, anorexia, hallucinations, numbness and tingling of extremities, headache, memory loss, seasonal affective disorder, muscle/leg cramps, confusion, nervousness, and disorientation. This is by no means an exhaustive list, but it certainly is exhausting just to think about! My point is, no matter how hard we try, our lifestyles often lead to erratic diets. We can't strictly control the quality, sources, or management of our food. And having PCOS makes you even more sensitive to deficiencies and imbalances.

Additionally, some of the medications commonly taken by women with PCOS, particularly birth control pills and metformin, can contribute to deficiencies. Other medications that may affect your vitamin and mineral levels include Orlistat (over-the-counter name Alli, that fun one that makes fat slide through your body and has "loose, oily stools" listed among its side effects), antibiotics, diuretics (commonly used for blood pressure control), anticonvulsants (a psychotropic medication in some cases), and corticosteroids. Alcoholism, too much zinc (those popular throat lozenges), too much sugar, and overly processed foods are other contributors to deficiency.

When I first meet with a client, I always ask when she last had a physical check-up. It's important to have current blood work to rule out thyroid imbalances, check for diabetes, and assess for Vitamin D deficiency (remember, Vitamin D is a hormone, and we're all about hormones here). But beyond that, your doctor isn't likely to be testing for vitamin and mineral deficiencies. Some of this may be trial and error, or common sense, but please remember that it IS possible to overdo it with supplementation, or to create a new imbalance by over-supplementing with certain vitamins and minerals. Some alternative healthcare practitioners offer testing for vitamin and mineral deficiencies, but this is not typically covered by insurance, and may not be reliable.

If this feels overwhelming, I suggest finding a qualified practitioner such as an integrative registered dietician, functional medicine doctor, or naturopathic doctor, who really understands and applies the principles of supplementation correctly. You don't need to see them weekly for the rest of your life, but a few meetings to outline goals and priorities, and get some more education, may be one of the best things you can do for your health. The other reason it's important to not just take a random approach is that there's often a lot of detective work involved in getting your supplementation correct. Sometimes a small variation in dosage, source, or administration can really make a difference. While recommending specific supplements or dosing is outside the scope of my practice, I will share the most common dosage recommendations.

Ideally, you will identify a holistic and integrative psychiatrist, nutritionist, acupuncturist, or other doctor to make recommendations for your over-the-counter supplements. Proceed with caution when consulting people who have a vested interest in selling you their products, those who may have limited scientific education or meaningful professional credentials (such as personal trainers or the staff at a health food store). While it's rare to cause damage with herbs or supplements, it certainly is possible. I also suggest doing your own research from reputable sources on the internet before committing to taking anything new. Because research and professional opinions are always changing, this list is almost surely incomplete. At the same time, the list is so long that I opted to include it in alphabetical order in the book's *Appendix: Supplements for PCOS Brain Health,* along with the most salient information for PCOS patients.

Here are my favorite five PCOS brain health supplements:

- Magnesium for mood and cortisol regulation.
- Zinc helps to activate GABA receptors.
- GABA for anxiety reduction.
- Sam-E to improve depression.
- Turmeric to reduce inflammation/provides mild antidepressant effect.

Other Non-Prescription Treatment Options

In addition to herbs and supplements, there are other treatments that are available without a prescription. These include light therapy, massage therapy, meditation, and weighted blankets.

Light Boxes/Light Therapy can be valuable for treating depression, and there are several ways to use light for mood improvement. The easiest method is to simply go outside when it's sunny, 20 to 30 minutes per day. Another option is a dawn simulator used with your bedroom light(s), which mimics naturally occurring early morning light patterns. If you opt for a light box, you sit in front of an inexpensive home use machine that emits light for 15 to 30 minutes. Some studies show that light therapy has an equivalent effectiveness to antidepressants, but do not stop taking an antidepressant without consulting a physician first. Your psychiatrist or therapist may have a recommendation for a particular brand or treatment schedule.

Extreme caution should be utilized with light therapy if you have been diagnosed with, or suspect you have, bipolar disorder. A mixed state or hypomania may be triggered or worsened. Light therapy may also pose problems if you are taking St. John's Wort, tricyclic antidepressants, or certain prescription medications, so do your research.

I am not a morning person, so I tend to miss the sunlight and get some mood symptoms in the winter. I like to use a light box during that time of year, for 20 minutes while I am doing my morning meditation.

Massage therapy is the manual manipulation of muscles, tendons, ligaments, and fascia to reduce stress, improve circulation, and enhance overall well-being. It is typically performed with you fully undressed, or undressed "to your comfort." There are many forms of massage, ranging from very soft to deep and hard. Some are more for pleasure and relaxation while others are designed to reprogram movement patterns or provide release from pain. Massage may be performed by licensed or unlicensed massage therapists, reflexology studios, chiropractors, or physical therapists. I find massage to be a good stress and tension reducer and try to get one at least once a month.

There are a number of cautions. You should not get a massage if you are sick with something contagious, vomiting, have diarrhea, are in severe pain, or have open wounds or sores. Cancer patients should always consult with their doctors before obtaining massage therapy. I also advise proceeding with caution if you have a history of sexual trauma, as it can trigger uncomfortable memories. If you wish to try it anyway, you could start with a massage where you remain clothed, such as a shiatsu massage.

Meditation is fully described in *Chapter 16: Developing a Meditation Practice.*

Weighted blankets emerged as a calming treatment for patients with autism spectrum disorders and other sensory processing disorders and have gone mainstream with applications for anxiety, insomnia, and other mental health disorders. The blankets can be laid across your lap, wrapped around your shoulders, or used to cover your entire body. Some people with travel anxiety take them in the car or on the plane. There are also weighted vests, socks, etc. The pressure (specifically deep touch pressure) from the weight releases serotonin and endorphins in the body, which is soothing. They may be weighted with charcoal, pewter, stone, or pellets made of various materials. Recommendations for weights are 5% to 10% of one's ideal body weight, with a commonly used formula being 10% of body weight plus a pound or two. They are commercially available and a little expensive, but I've had good reports from a number of clients, and I am all for non-pharmaceutical approaches to providing relief or healing.

There are many, many other supplements, vitamins, herbs, and proprietary blends that are not addressed here, but may be helpful for sleep, menstrual regulation, depression, anxiety, and other mood disorders. If you are curious, you might research some of the ones I think may be useful for other aspects of PCOS: selenium, ginseng, wild yam, cramp bark, yarrow, mugwort, peppermint, spearmint, black cohosh, borage oil, gingko, chamomile, passionflower, and saffron.

In sum, I do not believe that western medicine adequately addresses the complexity of PCOS with its standard pharmaceutical prescriptions. It is my experience that a mix of pharmaceutical and "natural" or alternative remedies yields the best long-term health results. I've also consulted with many women with PCOS who experiment heavily on themselves with various herbs, supplements, and alternative treatments. Responses are highly individualized, and it may take a lot of experimentation to find what works for you. The "magic formula" that works for me may do nothing for you. What gives me a side effect may give you bliss. And what calms me down may hype you up.

It's important to take a measured approach to experimentation. In other words, don't go out and add eight new supplements to your life all in one day. You won't know which one of those is giving you either benefits or unwanted side effects. You need to be patient, thorough in your research, and careful – and preferably able to work with a skilled practitioner who can help monitor and guide you.

If mixed with other supplements (for example, if you're playing around with Chinese herbs, Native American herbs, and Ayurvedic herbs at the same time), you may unwittingly increase the chance of negative reactions. While these types of supplements are not regulated in the same way that prescription medications are, they are powerful medications nonetheless. I recommend working with a licensed professional, particularly a holistic and integrative psychiatrist.

In the next chapter, we'll begin looking at ways to improve your mental health by building life skills by getting proactive, practicing acceptance, managing anger, dealing with pain, developing a meditation practice, improving sleep, and exercising for health.

Key Takeaways from This Chapter

- Vitamins, minerals, and amino acids are necessary for good brain functioning and repair.
- Adaptogens may be particularly helpful for women with PCOS.
- Whole foods are the best sources of the nutrients you need.
- It's difficult to get all the nutrients if you are following a strict vegan or vegetarian diet.
- Women with PCOS may have numerous insufficiencies and imbalances that can be improved by selective supplementation.
- Five of my favorites for mental health are: GABA, turmeric, magnesium, zinc, and Sam-E.
- Always start slowly with supplementation and consult with a health professional for dosing advice.

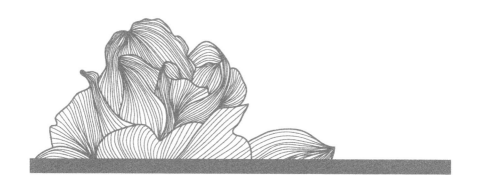

Part Three:
PCOS Life Skills

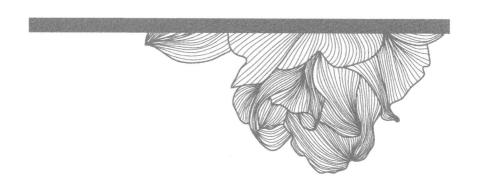

CHAPTER 12
Getting Proactive

Women with PCOS consistently have more stress in their bodies and brains than other people. This means that you need to address any underlying emotional and psychological issues that are consuming energy and focus in your life so that you can devote yourself to developing better health practices. Dealing with any underlying issues that are throwing you off balance will allow you to focus on developing your strengths and becoming more proactive in developing a long-term strategy for self-care. I emphasize being *proactive*, because being *reactive* to your PCOS will tend to lead to frustration, panic, wasted time and money, and a worsened disease state overall.

So, what one needs are healthy coping skills, defined as an ability to deal *effectively* with the stressors that life presents. A stressor is simply a person, place, or situation that creates stress (which can be good or bad stress, by the way). When you forget to pay the phone bill on time, there's a last-minute call for cupcakes for your child's class party, or a family member has to go to the emergency room, your coping skills get called into play. Your resources are even more taxed when the stressors are greater, such as a death in the family, diagnosis of illness, or a job loss. Dealing effectively doesn't necessarily mean getting what you want; it means achieving a workable solution and having adequate acceptance of and knowledge about a situation to make good decisions.

Everyone needs good coping skills, but the woman with PCOS needs them far more than average, because I think we can all agree that PCOS is a situation and a half! If you don't already have good coping skills, this is something you can learn by practicing. Yes, coping skills can be learned! There's a mindset and basic approach that I find very helpful in learning how to deal with stress effectively, briefly outlined here, and more fully described below.

Skills and Techniques for Managing Stress

Practice acceptance. Accept stress as an inevitability and a normal part of daily life. Remember that acceptance is different from giving up. Acceptance is understanding the challenges, knowing the downsides, and knowing that you have done your best by calling on your support system, your knowledge, and your internal strength - doing the things you know you need to do, and giving yourself credit for doing your best in this moment. Refer to *Chapter 12: Practicing Acceptance* for more details.

Be proactive. Author Peter McWilliams, who wrote a number of well-known books including, *How to Survive the Loss of a Love,* defined a victim as "a person to whom life happens." How about being "a person who happens to life?" I believe that getting assertive about your health and well-being contributes to feelings of self-esteem and efficacy. In other words, it will make you feel better about yourself, just by trying, even if you don't find the kind of outcome you're looking for initially.

Context stress in the grand scheme of the world and adjust the level of importance. Use a 10-point scale to assess stress. For example, when it's immediate and personal, stress may feel intense: getting in a fender-bender on the freeway may feel like a 10. But when you look at it broadly, it's probably a five on that 10-point scale, and maybe less if you've got good insurance.

Set realistic goals. If your to-do list always has 12 items on it, and you routinely only complete six of them, it's time to reconsider your goals. Consider surrendering to the fact that six items are all you can do. If you reduce the list to something realistic, you can end your day feeling productive rather than like you've failed. Routinely setting goals that exceed your ability to meet them results in disappointment, frustration, anger, and sometimes worse, especially in the job setting.

Prepare for stress in advance. Be reasonable, not obsessive. Having a strategy tends to reduce stress. By keeping a well-organized calendar, setting requirements for the other people in your life (including children, spouses, and colleagues) to keep you informed of events that affect you, and making a concerted effort to build adequate time into your daily schedule, you'll be able to more easily incorporate the surprises with grace.

Remember that women with PCOS feel stress more quickly and more intensely than women who don't have PCOS. Stress creates endocrine shifts, as well as mood shifts. It's up to you to know this and plan for it accordingly. It's so much better to tell your boss you'll submit a project on Thursday, and then be able to turn it in on Wednesday, than the other way around.

Redefine failure and success. Success and failure are actually very personal concepts. It's up to you to define them in ways that support you, rather than make you feel bad about yourself. Instead of defining weight loss success as getting down to a size six, perhaps you could redefine it as fitting into the next size down, being able to bend over to tie your shoes easily, or losing 12 pounds in the space of a year. *To maintain a positive focus on your progress, keep a daily written record of the things you did to support your health and self-care goals. Updating the list daily will soon show you how much you actually are doing, and this should feel really good.*

Learn new skills. The more you know, the less stressful things seem. You may be great at setting up a spreadsheet and lousy at getting dinner on the table five nights a week. Take a cooking class, buy a book on batch cooking, or get the more interested, talented, or available individuals in your life to take over the task. Or perhaps you are good at standing up to clients who demand too much, and not so good at standing up to your in-laws. Take an assertiveness training class or see a therapist who can help you develop these skills. Almost any problem you have managing your life has a corresponding expert who is willing to train you in how to improve your effectiveness.

Get educated. Do some research on the internet, ask your doctor a lot of questions, join a support group like my PCOS Psychology page on Facebook and use it, read the RESOLVE infertility newsletter, log in regularly to chat rooms on PCOSChallenge.com, and stay on top of developments in treatment. An educated mind is a powerful mind. I always say that the patient is the expert on her own body and mind; I am merely a guide. Since you're the expert, you have to educate others about the details of what's going on with you, and what your experience is. Just because you've got PCOS doesn't mean that anyone else really knows what it means. There are many different presentations of PCOS physically and emotionally. Even other patients don't necessarily know what you mean, unless you detail it for them. Tell them what it means for you and see if things change. The more you help people to understand you, the better they're able to respond, and the better you feel about the relationship.

Have a back-up plan. Back-up plans make life so much easier when life goes awry, as it so often does. Know who you can call, how you're going to pay, what an alternate route looks like, how late you can submit the document, etc. Have a frozen meal ready for times when you don't have time to even stop by a restaurant. Go through your outfits on Sunday, making sure you have enough clean and appropriate clothes for all the activities in the upcoming week. Buy a few extra all-purpose cards and gifts and keep them tucked away for birthdays. That way, when the stress of daily life hits, you are ready, and when the bigger stressors arrive, you don't have to worry about the smaller things.

Individualize the plan. What works for someone else might not work for you. If I've got adequate battery on my smart phone, I don't feel like I need to print out all my travel itineraries; maybe you feel better having a paper file.

Break things down into smaller pieces so they look less overwhelming. Work on just one piece at a time. Most meaningful projects feel overwhelming at the beginning. When you can do this, the project or situation starts to look more manageable.

Challenge assumptions – yours and others. Maybe you don't need to show up before dinner to set-up, or bring an artisan dessert, or read the entire book before you write the paper. Learning how to gently reduce expectations and redefine success helps to reduce stress.

Maybe have another back-up plan! I'm a big believer in at least thinking things through in advance, even if you don't map out a formal plan. Knowing in advance what you're willing to compromise on is also helpful.

Line up your support team. Again, have a first choice (your boyfriend, your best friend, your mom) and a second choice, like another friend or acquaintance, or a colleague. If you have a spiritual belief or practice, add that to your list of supports as well.

Work on building even more supportive relationships. As women, we are relational, and operate best within an extensive web of support. If you've been neglecting your friendships, give them some immediate attention. It's not a one-shot deal though; you've got to continuously provide time and attention. Strengthening relationships now gives you a place to turn later, if you need it. Besides, you'll have a lot more fun along the way! If you have few or no friends, have recently moved or changed schools or jobs, or just wish you knew more people, start investigating meet up groups in your area, cultural and religious organizations, neighborhood organizations, etc. Proximity and frequency are necessary components to building relationships.

Seek outside help. Whether it be professional therapy, time with a yoga teacher, membership in a support group, or a return to a spiritual practice, seek help. The advice and wisdom of others is invaluable in supporting your decision-making process. Decisions feel better when they're backed-up with the experience of others. And again, I want to emphasize that knowledge is power when it comes to PCOS. With so few reliable official sources of information, it becomes even more important to find people who share the same experience so that you can gather new tips, share your experiences, and receive support. Contributing in return also feels good.

Maintain an optimistic outlook. Studies repeatedly show that those who maintain an optimistic outlook have a higher perceived rate of life satisfaction. Maintaining optimism means keeping your eyes open for opportunities, positive moments, and the hidden benefits of what's stressing you out. Whether it's perception or reality, the bottom line is, you feel better when you stay positive.

Challenge #5: List Five Positive Things About PCOS

If it seems impossible, try harder! I'll give you a few freebies:

- You're getting proactive about your health at a time in life when others are still partying and acting like they're never going to get old.
- Accessing a community of women with PCOS is easier than ever, with resources like PCOS Wellness, PCOS Challenge, and Facebook.
- Gaining a deep understanding of your biochemistry and mood is a great way to manage your relationships more effectively; you *know* why you're cranky or sad.

Adjust accordingly and keep repeating as needed.

Additional Skills for Getting Proactive About Your Body

Obtain skilled medical help. Although an internist or general practitioner may diagnose PCOS, it is more likely that a gynecologist, endocrinologist, or reproductive endocrinologist will do so. If you have PCOS, you will most likely want to have an endocrinologist who will prescribe appropriate medications, monitor you for diabetes, and coordinate with your reproductive endocrinologist if you are trying to get pregnant. Because women with PCOS experience higher rates of thyroid disorders and heart disease, it is a good idea to have frequent monitoring. Your physician can also:

- Help you lose weight with the assistance of certain medications, and/or referral to a skilled dietician, who can teach you how to eat in a way that contributes to balancing your hormones and managing your symptoms.

- Refer you to a good dermatologist, who can help to control or eliminate skin conditions related to PCOS, such as skin darkening (acanthosis nigricans), acne, and hair loss.
- Suggest a therapist or support group to help you cope with the stress of infertility, symptoms of depression and frustration of dealing with a chronic disease.

For more on this topic, take a look at *Chapter 8: Assembling Your PCOS Health Team.*

Exercise. You've heard it before, and I'll tell you again – walking is one of the best things you can do for your body. *Chapter 18: Exercising for Health* explores this topic in detail. Thirty minutes a day helps regulate insulin levels, exposes you to the energetic benefits of the sun, and helps you focus on something other than your work or home stressors. Walking is one of the best ways to regulate PCOS-related insulin resistance and control weight. The cross-lateral motion of walking is also highly effective at resynchronizing your brain waves. I also am a huge fan of yoga for virtually every medical and mental health condition. It will reset your brain, produce deep relaxation, reduce stress, and enhance body acceptance. There are many classes available online, at most gyms, and in private studios in most communities. Look for beginner's classes, yoga for relaxation, or "curvy yoga" when you're starting. As long as you have no physical reason not to engage in exercise, there's not much downside to walking or yoga.

In addition, anything else you can do that counts as movement is great – dancing, Pilates, swimming, running, cycling, even gardening – it all adds up. You undoubtedly know the benefits for weight management, but more importantly, exercise makes you feel good in your body. As you develop strength, agility, and endurance, you'll also develop confidence and a greater sense of comfort and belief in the capacities of your body and mind to prevail.

Look better so you feel better: In addition to seeking the help of a dermatologist for skin and hair conditions, you might want to actively manage excess hair growth cosmetically. Temporary methods include plucking, waxing, and shaving. Laser hair removal takes several sessions, but is effective for those who have dark hair on light skin. Electrolysis is the only method that has been proven permanent. A licensed electrologist will have a great deal of experience with PCOS patients. Your dermatologist can provide you with a safe and reliable referral.

Although weight gain around the middle is frustrating and hard to overcome when you have PCOS, you can learn how to dress well, no matter your size or shape – and you deserve to do so! Seek out current fashions that are figure-friendly and get help when you need it. If you're just not good at putting outfits together, ask a friend who is good at it to go shopping with you, help you clear out your closet, or make some outfits that you can take pictures of for reference. You can also use the free services of a department store personal shopper, look through a bunch of style books or pictures on Pinterest, or spring for a professional stylist who will help you figure out what works on you. The difference that results in feeling like you look your best is amazing. And the benefit that comes with feeling good is a tendency to get out and socialize more, which improves your mental health. Fashion isn't frivolous at all!

Strengthening Your Mind and Spirit

Remember your brain. Education is only one element of what your mind needs to effectively cope with the effects of PCOS. Sometimes friends, partners, and physicians aren't quite enough to help you work through your anger, frustration, irritability, and sadness about having PCOS, not being able to get pregnant, or the difficulty you experience losing weight despite eating well and exercising regularly. A licensed psychotherapist can help you decrease stress, develop personalized coping methods, enhance your support group, and identify additional resources. Many therapists use mind/body methods that include meditation, guided visualization, mindfulness, and other ways of supplementing your good health practices.

By actively taking care of your physical and mental health and appearance, you can learn to feel better by knowing that you are doing the best you can with a challenging condition. By anticipating challenges, you can be better prepared to handle them. With these skills in place, you will be able to handle most of life's stressors with grace, and perhaps a little humor.

Address your grief. This is really important because grief is often overlooked and may lead to feelings of anxiety, depression, sadness, and lethargy. You might need to grieve your fertility, your sexuality, your health, your beauty, the ability to eat freely and recklessly, or any number of other things. Why not try making a list of what makes you feel sad when you think about PCOS? That will give you a very good idea of what it is that needs to be grieved.

Practice gratitude. The more you focus on the positive, the more you squeeze out the negative. It's as simple as that. Try keeping a gratitude journal. Every day, list five to 10 things you're grateful for. Then increase it to 20 things, for example. You might be amazed how much you really do have to feel grateful for.

Indulge yourself. Not with unhealthy foods or designer purses, but by buying yourself the best you can afford. Purchasing quality services, supplements, medical care, books, and organic food allows you to say: "I tried my hardest, I worked with the best I could manage, and so, I really have done as well as I can." Knowing the truth of that is very satisfying.

Become a PCOS advocate or educator. This is an advanced coping skill, and it's not suitable for everyone, so don't feel like you have to do it, or your mental health will be compromised. Becoming a PCOS educator or activist will help you feel empowered while you are empowering other women with PCOS to get healthier, obtain good services, and prioritize the well-being of all women. You can do this in simple ways (signing a petition, posting something about PCOS on Facebook) or more time-consuming ways (giving a speech, writing a letter to your Congress person, or going to see him/her in person).

Practice positive thinking. The power of positive thinking is legendary. What you give energy to grows. I know it can be difficult to summon up positive energy, but there are many ways to get help with this. Share your experiences with an optimistic and supportive friend. Read a daily meditation book. Check out websites that are both supportive and proactive, such as PCOS Wellness, and participate in helping someone else out with information or your experience. Watch or listen to something that makes you laugh on a regular basis. All these things will help improve your mood and attitude.

Make positive choices. Emotions are a choice, so make positive choices. I'm not saying to deny the emotions, but once you've acknowledged them, let them go. It's not about not having "negative" emotions, but rather, about focusing on emotions that are more positive, uplifting, resourceful, galvanizing, etc. If you are feeling stuck in an unpleasant emotion, it is helpful to formally limit the amount of time you allow yourself to be stuck in negativity. You can set a timer on it and do it full-on – be angry, be resentful, be pessimistic or cranky. And then stop when the timer goes off. Bonus points if you can laugh at your bad mood after you do this.

Practice mindfulness. You've probably heard the term "mindfulness" and wondered exactly what that means. One of the most noted practitioners of mindfulness, Jon Kabat-Zinn, defines mindfulness as: "Paying attention in a particular way: on purpose, in the present moment, and non-judgmentally." Mindfulness is trendy now, but it's actually an ancient concept that is well supported by scientific research. It's free, easy to learn, and highly effective. It's not a cure-all for everything that ails you, but it's quite helpful as a coping skill, especially when it comes to quieting anxiety, and working with eating-disordered behavior. And since it's so easy to learn, I'm going to teach you right now. *Chapter 16: Developing a Meditation Practice* goes into this with much more depth. Is there a catch? Well, yes, it's easy to learn and much harder to practice, but the results are well worth it.

In its simplest form, mindfulness might apply to a behavior like slowing down enough to make a conscious action about something – say, cheesecake versus a pear. Or sitting with your fear for a moment, recognizing it, and then not snapping at someone in anger. Key components of mindfulness include maintaining a single focus and staying in the present.

Multi-tasking is the opposite of mindfulness, because your mind isn't focused on anything exclusively. You may think you're being more efficient, but you're actually being less efficient. We all do it: working on your laptop while watching television, applying makeup while eating breakfast and keeping one eye on the news, or half-listening to your spouse while reading the paper. We do these things so often, we forget that we're not actually paying attention. When our attention is consistently divided, we develop chronic low-level anxiety. On the other hand, practicing mindfulness has been shown to reduce anxiety, alleviate depression, and increase attention and concentration. In fact, even just practicing mindfulness regularly for a few weeks has been found to rewire your brain and increase your gray matter. Since most women with PCOS already feel more anxious than other people, you can see how so-called multi-tasking would just compound the problem.

Staying present-focused will help reduce your stress and make you more productive. Stop thinking about your grocery list while you're making love, or about how you want your own baby when you're attending someone else's baby shower. Don't let the sad experiences of the past take over the present moment. If this is challenging, a simple mindfulness meditation practice will help. Close your eyes. Breathe in deeply for a count of four. As you inhale, visualize oxygen moving through your respiratory system and imagine any stress you've been holding float away. Then exhale for a count of eight. Repeat five times. There are numerous other mindfulness meditations available at meditation groups, yoga studios, and online. Check resources in the back of the book for additional information.

Learn the art of the reframe. Reframing is a technique used to shift from a negative perspective to a more optimistic perspective. Simply put, the frame is our beliefs and experiences. Reframing is about flipping your experience in the moment. You can apply reframing to almost any subject or experience:

- My client cancelled; that's a bummer OR great, now I have time to respond to email!
- Life is really hard OR the universe gives me amazing challenges, and I meet them.
- Losing my uterus meant loss of my femininity OR losing my uterus means I regained my health.

Challenge #6: Try a Reframing Exercise

Write down five negative thoughts that come into your mind regularly and try reframing them as described above. It will feel awkward at first, but like any skill, it improves with practice. It's not about being unrealistic or denying what's going on; it's about choosing to see and handle it differently. Same experience; different perspective. Try it. It's powerful. Using a proactive approach to manage your PCOS will also have amazing, positive effects on the rest of your life.

CHAPTER 13
Practicing Acceptance

When you ask women about their PCOS, and how/when they developed it, you'll hear a wide range of answers, from "I was born with it and have lived with it all my life, so it's part of me," to "I don't know," to "when I hit puberty," or "when I tried to get pregnant and couldn't." I think the truth is, we ARE born with the genes that manifest as PCOS, but the symptoms typically don't start to appear until puberty.

Symptoms may be subtle, confusing, or go undiagnosed for a long time, if ever. Consequently, women with PCOS have a wide range of experiences when it comes to dealing with their condition. It may be something that feels almost like nothing except for one or two pesky symptoms, or it may be the focus of a woman's life. In particular, if a woman is trying to get pregnant, it's going to be a huge focal point in her life, as well as the life of her spouse or partner. Some of us blow it off and act like we don't care, some of us deny that it exists at all, and some of us use it as the excuse for every bad behavior or bad attitude you can imagine.

There's a huge range of ways of coping with PCOS styles; some of them are more effective than others. Also, there are times in a woman's life when PCOS is just going to require more attention. When you get some other diagnosis, go to a new doctor, discover new information on the internet, or get angry about it and activated enough to do something, all of a sudden, you're focused on it. All of that can be healthy.

Like anything else, there's a sequence to coping with PCOS. A lot of times, it looks like this:

- I have weird or unexplained symptoms.
- I do an internet search of my symptoms and make a self-diagnosis.
- I go see a doctor, or two, or three anyway, just for confirmation.
- I get an official PCOS diagnosis.
- I get upset and learn something about how to reduce my symptoms.
- I go on a diet, start exercising, and start taking one or more prescriptions.
- I feel better.
- I get tired of following a low glycemic diet, exercising like a maniac, taking drugs, or going for laser hair treatments.
- I get frustrated and angry.
- I tell my friends and anyone else who will listen.
- I go on a chat board and complain about it.
- Other women with PCOS validate me.
- I get over it.
- I decide to stop making PCOS the center of my life.
- I figure I have learned how to "cope" effectively.

Problem solved in a mere 15 steps, right?! Until…the diet stops working, you turn 40 and your doctor sends you to a cardiologist, a new doctor tells you that you wouldn't be fat if you just stopped eating so much, you have to add a second medication for insulin resistance or even diabetes, you can't get pregnant, or any of a number of situations. Then you start the cycle all over again, as you look for more answers, or a better answer. It's all utterly exhausting.

What if There Was a Better Way to Live With PCOS?

Let's look at two very different case examples, both women with PCOS:

Case Example, Delrio:

> Delrio was a woman with an office manager job, working for a bunch of workaholic consultants who wanted her to come in on the weekends, work through lunch, revise meeting documents literally as the meeting attendees were walking in the door – and that was just their usual behavior. On bad days, they'd leave her voice-mail messages that went on for 60 minutes or more, listing things for her to do. She was a conscientious employee, but it was overwhelming. One day, Delrio found herself in tears, hiding out in an empty office crying, under the desk (yes, on the floor) in case someone walked in. She followed up the cry with a giant bag of potato chips and was planning on at least one large cocktail when she got home. She felt like she was having a nervous breakdown, and in fact, ended up taking a psychiatric leave of absence for a month to rebalance herself. Delrio definitely could have used some help.

Now let's look at a different woman:

Case Example, Annabeth:

> Annabeth had a similar job to Delrio's – lots of responsibility, and not a lot of pay, involving keeping the office functions going. Her bosses were less insensitive than Delrio's, but she had far more of them, and they often made conflicting demands on her time. But Annabeth was really proactive in managing her PCOS and had even gone to see a therapist for help. She was learning how to use diet, exercise, meditation, and other skills to reduce her stress.

With the approval of her boss, Annabeth instituted a written system of work requests that included a priority and urgency rating. People who cried wolf and created chaos for Annabeth were quickly identified and dealt with by the boss. Annabeth was able to track her progress, document that she was meeting goals, and identify problematic projects and timeframes early on. Although this tracking system sounds complex, it actually simplified her work life a great deal. Each day, she knew pretty much what to expect. And on those occasions when things got really busy, she reminded herself that, in the grand scheme of things, most of what she was doing would be pretty meaningless in the space of a year's time. This perspective kept her from feeling an internal pressure on top of the external pressure. She was still under-paid, but at least Annabeth wasn't stressed to the point of tears. She actually felt calm, in control, and productive. Annabeth is an example of using great coping skills.

Learning how to manage PCOS starts with some basic skills that I outline in this book. It helps to start with acceptance, then address the underlying emotional and psychological issues and follow-up with a proactive long-term strategy for managing the condition. If you're thinking "shouldn't a doctor be creating the strategy for me," my response is an emphatic NO. That's giving your power away and falling victim to PCOS. I believe in strong, smart women (that's you, in case you were wondering!) taking consistent action to manage PCOS so that PCOS doesn't manage them.

Acceptance is not just saying "yeah, yeah, I've got PCOS," but really owning it, feeling it, and knowing it deeply. It's part of you that cannot be escaped. You can spend your whole life fighting it or pretending it's not there, or it's not that bad, or you can dig in and make the most of your life and your body. This is a far better approach than ignoring PCOS because PCOS is a really insidious condition that can cause all sorts of harm at different points in your life.

Acceptance has become a buzzword, a prescription for healing virtually every crisis of mind and body, and a general irritant to those of us who are not inclined to just shut up and accept the status quo. Nonetheless, it's important to go through the steps to get to the point of true acceptance. When I say "true acceptance," I mean the kind of acceptance that brings you some peace, not the kind that leaves you in a constantly alternating state of rage and despair about your PCOS. It's deeper than saying "yeah, great, now I've got this lousy diagnosis, *I accept it,* fix me so I can get on with my life." To get to acceptance, you will probably go through some anger. Since most of us aren't used to expressing our anger freely, this might be a challenging task. You will also need to spend time thinking about what PCOS means to you, and how it changes your plan for your life. *What does it mean to not be entirely in control of your body, your mind, and your existence?*

When I think about acceptance, I think about Elizabeth Kubler-Ross, who was famous for her work with terminally ill patients. In the 1960s, she created a process model commonly known as DABDA, which stands for Denial, Anger, Bargaining, Depression, and Acceptance. Over the years, it's been broadly applied to people who have lost a family member, and for many other situations in which grief seems appropriate. To get to acceptance of your PCOS diagnosis, you will probably go through DABDA.

The process of arriving at acceptance, whether of chronic illness, terminal illness, death, or some other hardship, is a complex, non-time-bound, non-linear process that weaves in and out of the DABDA stages. We really can't predict how long it's going to take someone to get through this process. It could take many years or appear to be over almost as quickly as it started. It's not helpful to compare yourself to others. In fact, it's probably detrimental, because comparing yourself to someone else who you think of as being more advanced in her process is bound to lead to feelings of shame, failure, and low self-worth – and who wants that? With PCOS, acceptance is a state you may move in and out of with some frequency, depending upon what's happening for you medically or psychologically. If you read *Gretchen's Story* at the beginning of this book, you probably noticed my moving in and out of acceptance and denial throughout the years. I am a pretty typical PCOS patient in that way.

The stages or emotions you go through can occur repeatedly, out of order, in long phases, in short bursts, or not at all (for example, some skip depression, or bargaining). It's helpful to know what to look for though, so you can keep an eye on the end goal of acceptance, acceptance being the opposite of denial.

Denial

PCOS denial might sound something like:

- I don't have PCOS.
- PCOS is no big deal.
- It's not PCOS – it's something else they haven't figured out yet.
- I'll outgrow it.
- Having a baby will fix it.
- Having a hysterectomy will fix it.
- It doesn't matter, because I'm not trying to get pregnant.
- Those medications don't really work.
- If I take birth control pills, that will fix everything, right?

Anger

PCOS anger may be repressed, expressed directly or passively, or get diverted into:

- Eating whatever you want, whenever you want, regardless of what it does to your body or your mood.
- Refusing to exercise, practice meditation, or do other self-care practices.
- Acting out – overspending, overeating, unhealthy sexual behavior, doing drugs, drinking too much.
- Developing other stress-related illnesses.
- Being verbally or emotionally abusive towards spouse, kids, or others.

Bargaining

PCOS bargaining looks like this:

- Making a deal with God/god/the universe to be more attentive to him/her/it, if only the PCOS will go away.
- Over-exercising to compensate for eating badly.
- Eating badly but taking lots of medication or supplements to compensate for it.
- Figuring, "I'm young, I can do what I want until ____ age, then I'll behave."

Depression

PCOS depression merits an entire book of its own, but briefly, looks like:

- Sleeping too much or not enough.
- Eating too much or not nearly enough.
- Being irritable.
- Feeling suicidal.
- Feeling hopeless.
- Feeling helpless.
- Totally lacking initiative, motivation, or drive.
- Having a gloomy, pessimistic perspective on life.

Acceptance

PCOS acceptance looks like:

- Generally being pretty okay with what's going on, even when it's unpleasant.
- Eating, sleeping, and exercising appropriately (whatever you decide that means for you).
- Practicing good self-care in all aspects of your life.

- Having and using a stress reduction practice.
- Being grateful for what you do have.
- Being genuinely happy about the positives of your life.
- Treating others with kindness.
- Not constantly comparing yourself to others.

Now that you can see how the path to PCOS acceptance may be full of twists and turns and mixed up emotions, I hope that you'll feel more able to be patient with yourself. Direct the same kindness you would give to a friend who is struggling toward yourself as you navigate this. It will definitely make it easier. In the next chapter, I'm going to tackle one of the hardest parts: anger.

CHAPTER 14
Managing Anger

When it comes to PCOS, there is so much to be angry about I'm sometimes surprised that we PCOS patients are not all raging, all the time. At various times, you might experience anger towards:

- God, the universe, or some other higher power, because you have PCOS.
- Doctors, because they can't cure it, didn't diagnose it soon enough, won't run the tests you want, couldn't put the pieces together, or dismiss you too quickly.
- Your parents, because they gave you the genes that caused it, or didn't get you to a doctor soon enough, or took you to too many doctors.
- Any woman who doesn't have it.
- Men, because they can't have it (although it turns out this is not quite true, despite the fact that they have no ovaries!).
- The medical industry, because they haven't cured it either, they're moving too slowly, not enough providers are well-informed, etc.
- Your body, because it's not working "right" and that is NOT FAIR.
- Other people, for not understanding.
- Anyone who has children, if you want them.
- Anyone who seems to enjoy perfect health, despite living an obviously unhealthy lifestyle (like the daily consumer of fast food who still has a perfect cholesterol panel, and no weight issues).

- Yourself, for not doing your self-care better, more perfectly, or more often.
- Dieticians who tell you what to eat without understanding your particular brain chemistry, or insist that there's only one correct way to eat for PCOS.
- Any other medical professional, personal trainer, parent, friend, or other well-meaning individual you've ever encountered who said something stupid, irrelevant, pointless, misdirected, or even rude, in an effort to help you get your body to behave.

That's a pretty huge list, and it's undoubtedly not even a complete list. In fact, you should make your own list. *Pause right here and list everything that makes you angry about your PCOS.* We'll get back to that list later. You are absolutely right to have a lot of anger about a lot of things related to PCOS. But you can't live in anger all the time. Well, you can, but it's not a healthy choice.

So, how do you deal with all this anger, and get it out of your system, so you can move on to something more productive? And why do you even need to do that in the first place? I believe you need to get over the anger for the simple reason that, as the esteemed Sigmund Freud said, anger turned inward becomes depression, and we've already got enough trouble with that, given the hormonal set-up we're dealing with. Also, anger tends to lead to negativity, self-hatred, and a more pessimistic perspective, none of which is helpful in managing PCOS.

Physical Methods

You can get rid of your anger in a lot of ways. Journaling, talking to friends, and talk therapy are all great methods. Exercising your creativity may help as well. Creating collages, photographs, movies, music, or poetry that express your feelings are all great. I don't like to encourage violence, but some clients report that there can be some great satisfaction in doing things like playing those video games where things explode. But I do think it's important – really important – to get physical with your anger.

There's nothing more gratifying than releasing the energy that's pent up inside of you by:

- Taking old phone-books and throwing them in the garage or outside (or in some other space where you won't damage the furniture, walls, windows or, of course, other people). Throw them at the floor and the walls. Heave them and scream and huff and puff and talk to whomever/whatever you're angry at. Do this for three to five minutes. You will be stunned by how exhausting it is, and what a huge cathartic release you get.
- Screaming – not at another human being – but again, the garage is an excellent place, or the car's a great place for a little self-regulated primal scream therapy. Scream at the top of your lungs; you will feel a good release. Words are great; screaming without words is also great.
- Taking a boxing or kickboxing class. Do more than eyeball that heavy bag and slap it as you walk by. Learn how to hit correctly, or you'll injure yourself. Many gyms offer classes and personal trainers can show you the basics. This is sanctioned violence (and, oh yeah, it's ridiculously fun, plus you're burning a lot of calories without even thinking about it).
- Some sports, particularly those where you kick, throw, or catch something with a good satisfying thwack, like soccer, kick-ball, baseball, or softball may be a great way to get some anger out (imagine the ball is your PCOS, for example).
- Other sports with a hard, repetitive motion, like swimming, hitting a volleyball, tennis, or racquetball may also move this kind of energy. Focus your anger and use it to really drive the ball or the water.
- Hitting golf balls is great for this too – you can actually get away with grunting! Not a golfer? So what – rent a bucket of balls and borrow a club, and go at it anyway. Don't go out on the course because the "real" golfers will not be happy, but the driving range at most golf courses is free for anyone to use!

- Martial arts that are more combat-oriented, like karate, or Krav Maga may offer some aggressive elements that feel like a release of anger too. Sparring practice allows for an aggression and "attack" mode that shifts anger. Similarly, Model Mugging and other self-defense courses will teach you how to harness anger (and fear) and make it useful.

- Hitting soft stuff, like pillows, the couch, or the bed, with your hands, fists, another pillow, or a bataka (soft bat). Just be aware that this may frighten children, animals, and other members of your household, not to mention stir up a bunch of dust in your furniture. If you're really motivated by living green and practicing the old ways of housekeeping, find yourself a rug beater, haul a heavy rug outside, and beat it soundly – you'll have gotten rid of your anger and cleaned up the rug.

- Throwing crockery. As in ceramic dishes. This requires a little equipment and planning – cheap, breakable dishes or glassware (source garage sales and the dollar store – pick ugly ones so you won't feel guilty, or cull damaged items from your housewares, leftover tiles, etc.), some eye protection, long pants and long sleeves, and a safe place to do it – someplace with lots of space to safely bounce things around and shatter them. An empty commercial trash bin is excellent for this purpose. Get a stack of dishes and go for it – the sound is excellent, and quite satisfying. One creative friend of mine used a sharpie to write on plates before she broke them, like "my evil stepmother," "the teacher who failed me in seventh-grade history," etc., which added a nice therapeutic dimension to the exercise. Various unattractive gifts have also been known to end up as fodder for this sort of therapy activity (that vase your mother-in-law gave you? – I'm just saying' – whatever it takes, within reason).

- Pounding meat for a meal – there are many recipes calling for pounded chicken, pork, or beef cutlets. It really doesn't take long to do this, but if you've got a mallet and a cutting board, put it to good use. Also, you'll already be finished with step one of a healthy homemade meal.

- Hammering nails – again, this is about force, and focus. And, it can be a sort of meditative activity as well. It might even be useful if you've got some pictures to hang, or floorboards to repair.
- Breaking up stone, cement, or drywall for a home improvement project, doing some preliminary demolition of walls and counters, etc. Again, be mindful of safety and wear protective clothes and goggles. This stuff is fun, messy, and a great way to let go ("take that, you jerk who cut me off in traffic!"). It doesn't come along every day, unless you're in the construction biz, but when it does, it's a great opportunity to release some wild pent-up anger.

You get the idea. Anything that can be fast, furious, and forceful will be capable of helping you release anger, when done with focus and intention.

Journaling and Unsent Letters

If the physical methods don't appeal to you, or just aren't practical, you can get your anger out in writing too, either through journaling or use of "the unsent letter" technique.

Journaling is one of my favorite techniques for expressing emotions, exploring thoughts, and working through problems. Some people keep journals online, but I recommend keeping a handwritten journal. Handwriting forces you to slow down, and it activates neurons in your brain in ways that are similar to meditation. It doesn't matter if your handwriting is beautiful or sloppy, your spelling is perfect or frightful, or you're not much of a writer. This is not an artistic or literary exercise, unless you want it to be. Feel free to use different colors and sizes of pens, add drawings or collage in pictures, doodle designs, play with rhymes, etc. To give yourself even more freedom to play, I also recommend skipping the fancy, expensive handmade journals. Get a cheap lined notebook and experience the freedom of not filling those pages with perfect words and images.

Unsent letters are a favorite therapeutic homework assignment of mine. There is some overlap with journaling, but don't get uptight about keeping it in a category. Just write! You write a letter to the person, body part, institution, or whatever it is that you're angry at. Fully express yourself, complete with curse words and evil, destructive fantasies, if desired. And then shred the letter, burn the letter, or flush the letter. Similarly, the angry list you made at the start of this chapter can be shredded or burned with great satisfaction. As you destroy the list or letter, imagine all your anger disappearing along with the written words.

Here are some journaling and letter-writing prompts to get you started if you're feeling a little stuck or hesitant:

- List 15 things that make you smile.
- List all the things that you've changed in the past year.
- Create a bucket list.
- Write about your biggest and smallest talents.
- Describe the people in your life who are most supportive; what is it that makes their support so helpful?
- Describe what you're grateful for.
- What are some ways to nurture yourself when you're feeling down?
- What would you like to be remembered for?
- What makes you feel peaceful?
- If you went to live in another country, how would you be living differently? What can you change here and now to live more like this?
- How do you define true health?
- List 10 ways you know you're happy.
- How do you break out of a shame spiral?
- Write a letter to your teenaged self.
- Write a letter to your future self.
- What can you do to change your life or health?

You might find that your anger isn't just anger. Sometimes, you start out angry and end up crying. If you think you've got something to be sad about when it comes to PCOS, you're probably right. PCOS is a condition that adds the unwanted (facial hair, body fat, cardiac abnormalities, acne) and subtracts the desirable stuff (babies, the hair on your head, your sense of femininity). It's painful – really, deeply painful. But when you can shift the anger, you also get to move the sadness, which is part of the ultimate task of achieving real acceptance. By starting a conversation with your anger, you deepen an important connection to and within yourself. PCOS is a life altering experience; it's going to come with a whole lot of feelings.

Therapy

If none of this feels like enough, it's time to seek therapy. A licensed psychotherapist will help support and guide you safely into and through your anger, so that you can live a happier life that isn't constantly interrupted by angry outbursts and the depressed feelings that often go with anger.

CHAPTER 15

Dealing with Pain

There are many PCOS-related diagnoses that you're probably familiar with, like early onset type 2 diabetes, endometriosis, and cardiovascular disease. Chronic pain is a lesser known, but very common complaint for women with PCOS. Chronic pain is a problem that many clients report to me, but not until I ask. It turns out that not many doctors ask either, unless you come in specifically complaining of pain. When I ask, people often seem both surprised and relieved. I find that if it's something a woman's been dealing with for a long time, it's just become part of life. It's "normal," it seems untreatable, and so it becomes less of a focus than other problems. But pain is not normal. It's a message from your body that something is wrong and needs attention.

In addition to physical pain, you may be experiencing emotional, spiritual, or relational pain, all of which can worsen the experience of physical pain.

Physical Pain

You may have heard the antidepressant advertising tagline, "depression hurts," and the truth is, depression *does* hurt. It causes new physical pain and exacerbates existing physical pain. And chronic pain can also contribute to or cause depression. It's not uncommon for people with depression to report a lot more general aches and pains – things like headaches, neck aches, back aches, and other muscular aches. I've also observed an increased tendency in depressed patients to have more minor injuries, falls, cuts and bruises, or other sorts of pain. It appears that coordination is reduced in some depressed people, which makes sense when you consider the general slowing that is part of the overall condition. Having depression also makes it harder to cope with acute pain, as in the pain from an injury, or after surgery. The brains of people with depression are less able to fend off pain and, unfortunately, the more pain you have, the more difficult it seems to be to fight back against that pain. This sets up a terrible loop, which may feel inescapable and contribute to hopelessness.

It's important to address chronic pain to optimize your health. Treating chronic pain may require medical assessment and ongoing treatment, but it is most effectively treated when you work with a health psychologist or other professional who specializes in pain management techniques.

Pain is typically rated on a scale from zero or one to 10. If you've ever been in the hospital for any reason, you've probably used or noticed a pain-rating scale posted on the wall that includes "smiley faces" to indicate the degree of pain – you can simply point to the one that represents what you feel. Zero is no pain, and 10 is the worst pain imaginable. Although it's a self-rating scale, it's an important form of measurement. It lets professionals know what you need to feel better. It's obviously designed for physical pain, but it also works for other forms of pain, discomfort, or anxiety. You can rate your discomfort about almost anything, from your anxiety about going on a job interview to what your experience of stubbing your toe is like, by using a pain scale. It's a helpful reference point for your therapist too. Over time, you will develop a clearer sense of your pain, and what those ratings mean for you. If you're working with a professional, it's important to teach them what your scale means too – sometimes someone tells me they're at a seven, but I know them well enough to know that it would be a 10 on the average person's pain rating scale. That helps us figure out how to help you best.

Common Types of PCOS-Related Pain

The problem with pain, as it relates to PCOS, is that, while pain is not one of the diagnostic criteria for PCOS, there seems to be a lot of pain that goes along with PCOS. Some forms of pain you might experience include:

Mittelschmerz. From German, literally "middle pain" – this is the pain that occurs in your abdomen during ovulation, that sharp little ouch in your belly.

Endometriosis. When extra tissue deposits itself in your abdominal cavity, it can interfere not only with reproductive functions, but also penetrate or wrap itself around your bladder, bowels, and other organs. Endometriosis usually causes pain. Sometimes the pain seems to be for no apparent reason, and other times, if you're having a cycle, it seems to be linked to your cycle. You might also have pain from intercourse or medical examinations, such as pelvic ultrasound procedures, that are normally quite painless, if you have endometriosis.

Fibroids. Uterine fibroids are growths of smooth muscle and fibrous connective tissue in the uterus. They cause abnormal bleeding patterns and pain. They can grow as large as a six or seven-month pregnancy, and at that size, they press on other pelvic organs, sometimes even pushing them into another location in the abdomen.

Pre-Menstrual Syndrome. PMS can cause pain before and during your period, and the pain isn't confined to your abdomen. Many women report an increase in migraines and other forms of headache, leg cramps, and breast pain.

Pre-Menstrual Dysphoric Disorder (PMDD). This is a worse form of PMS that causes extreme mood swings and other debilitating psychological symptoms. The diagnostic criteria for PMDD include not only menstrual-type pain, but headaches, leg cramps, breast pain, and increased sensitivity to other pain.

Pain from cysts. Cyst-related pain can exist in women who don't have PCOS, but it's a routine occurrence for women with PCOS. It is normal to have some cysts, but women with PCOS may have an accumulation of cysts, or cysts that wrap around the ovaries or fallopian tubes, or become grossly enlarged within the ovaries. Sometimes these cysts are small, but they still cause pain when they spontaneously burst. Larger cysts can be extraordinarily painful, and even dangerous, if they burst, causing infection within the abdominal cavity which then requires antibiotic treatment or rarely, emergency surgery. There is also a tiny chance that a cyst may be cancerous. These potential complications often lead doctors to recommend surgical removal of cysts, which then leads to post-surgical pain – not forever, but as a typical after-effect of surgery.

Inflammation. Because PCOS is an inflammatory condition, and pain is also an inflammatory condition, other forms of chronic pain unrelated to PCOS may be exacerbated by PCOS pain.

Long-term pain isn't just annoying. It decreases immunity, leads to irritability and depression, and may cause or worsen insomnia, anxiety, and depression. It also leads to many lost work and school days. These are serious consequences. Pain negatively affects quality of life, and sometimes, desire to live. That's why it's important to take it very seriously. If your doctor or therapist doesn't ask about pain, please make sure to bring it up yourself.

Assessing Pain

To deal with pain effectively, we have to assess the problem completely. These are the sorts of questions that should be asked:

- Where is the pain?
- What is the quality of the pain (chronic, intermittent, intense, dull, sharp, diffuse, radiating, etc.)?
- What was going on when the pain started?
- How would you rate the intensity of pain?
- How long has the pain been there?
- What have you tried that relieves the pain?
- What have you tried that doesn't help?
- What aggravates the pain?
- How often does it occur?

- When does it occur?
- What time of day does it occur?

Pain management is a collaborative process, even more so perhaps than "just therapy." Long-term pain is wearing and frequently intolerable. It increases feelings of helplessness and hopelessness, key factors in depression. And it absolutely needs to be addressed as part of your mental health treatment plan. Rating and assessing your pain in consistent terms helps us make adjustments to optimize treatment as we progress. If we don't know what we're starting with, we don't know where we need to go, and we don't know when we have made progress. If something's not working, we can shift what we're doing and possibly get improvement more quickly.

Pain Management

Addressing pain issues is a multi-part (and multi-party) process. This is one reason it's so important for your health psychologist to work in coordination with your doctor. Some of the things that need to be addressed include:

- Discovering the underlying cause of your pain. This requires a medical evaluation to rule-out underlying issues, x-rays or other tests if appropriate, physical examination, and so on. Some physical pain, while quite strong, has no apparent physical cause. This can be quite frustrating for both the patient and the physician, and often results in a referral to a psychologist, on the assumption that the pain must be caused by a psychological problem. This may or may not be the case, but pain diagnoses are part of psychology, and health psychologists can definitely help with pain. The psychologist will probably go into more depth about the history of your pain, as well as the rest of your life, to develop a complete picture of the potential causes of your pain.

- Appropriate pain management techniques need to be applied. If it is clearly indicated for physical pain, these techniques will be prescribed by a physician, orthopedist, chiropractor, etc. They may include ice, heat, rest, physical therapy, massage, chiropractic manipulations, painkillers, steroids, anti-inflammatory medications, supportive braces, orthotics, or special shoes. Sometimes recommendations include surgery, depending upon the cause of the pain. Recovering from pain can be a slow process that requires a lot of time, attention, and follow-through on your part. Physical therapy, for example, will involve daily homework to get better.

- If you've had unresolved and/or unidentified pain for a long time, you may receive a referral to a pain management specialist. This is a physician who specializes in managing pain, particularly getting the right mix of medications that will relieve pain yet not result in addiction or dependency. They may also recommend physical therapy or working with a psychologist who will teach you relaxation exercises, stress management or stress reduction techniques, biofeedback practices, mindfulness, and other ways of reducing or eliminating pain.

- Development of a mindfulness practice can be quite helpful for a number of conditions, and pain is certainly one of them. Interestingly enough, you can actually reduce pain by shifting your focus to the pain, and allowing it to simply exist, and observing it, rather than trying to shove it out of your consciousness. I might even go so far as to say that buddying up to your pain and making friends with it can be informative and often leads to a reduction in pain.

- Gestalt therapy practices, including focusing on integration of the broken-off parts of the self, may also be helpful. Basically, what you reject or ignore continues to demand your attention. When you give it the attention that it needs, it may recede. In therapy, we give it appropriate attention. It stops nagging at you. You feel better.

- Physical exercise is often helpful in relieving pain too. Exercise releases endorphins, which make you feel good. If exercise is not contra-indicated by your condition (always, always, always clear it with your doctor first!), then it may help by increasing blood flow, releasing muscle constriction, and stimulating a sense of well-being. If your pain is caused or exacerbated by tension, as so much neck/back/shoulder pain and headache pain is, exercise may help alleviate the tension, thereby reducing your pain levels.

- Self-care practices in general are something that benefit people with pain issues. People who are working constantly and don't take breaks will have a lot more physical pain. If your work, school, or family life are highly stressful, you may also develop pain. Sometimes people don't know how to ask for a break, or demand better treatment in life, so they give themselves a break by developing pain, and making themselves disabled to varying degrees. That sounds strange, because who wants to be in pain, right? But it's more socially acceptable to be "sick" or injured than to admit to needing time, space, or rest. Therapy will uncover issues like this, if they're contributing to the pain.

- Dietary changes and targeted supplementation may also be helpful. There are many anecdotal reports of improvement in physical condition as a result of eating a healthier diet. That might simply be upping your intake of vegetables or eliminating wheat. Or it could be as complex as changing over to vegetarianism or doing an allergy elimination or rotation diet. Pain is an inflammatory condition, and many of the foods we eat can be inflammatory. I believe that dietary changes can definitely be helpful, especially if you have any sort of gastro-intestinal or pelvic pain, as well as diffuse joint pain. Women with hormonally-stimulated pain often report an improvement in symptoms by doing things like avoiding excessive caffeine, sodium, or sugar at relevant times of the month.

- Development of a spiritual practice may be helpful. It doesn't take the pain away, but having someone or something to pray to, talk to, blame, or seek answers from is supportive and meaningful for a lot of people. Try shifting the focus outside of yourself and your pain by turning it over to god or the universe.

- Work, or other purposeful, meaningful behavior or activities: I've observed that pain issues often increase when people are unemployed, become empty nesters, or have recently retired. That emptiness and lack of outer focus or sense of purpose may get somewhat distorted and become a focus on pain. If you can add purpose and focus to your life, even if it's not in a way that you're used to, you may find that your pain diminishes.

- Rest. I know, I just said work! On the flip side, an awful lot of us are just working far too many hours, with our butts planted behind a desk, or standing at a counter in the wrong shoes, or not taking days off or breaks throughout the day. Sitting or standing in one place for long periods often exacerbates pain. Old-school medical advice for back pain used to include rest, but now we know that movement is actually more beneficial. Consider what's causing your pain and see if rest might counter it. Those of you with hand, wrist, elbow, arm, neck and upper body pain – get off the keyboards now! And learn some stretches aimed at preventing carpal tunnel syndrome while you're at it. It could be as simple as saying, "this work is not as important right now as taking care of my body is."

- Support groups exist for virtually every diagnosis and problem. Many hospitals have support groups for people with pain issues. If the support group is competently led so that it offers support, as opposed to merely serving as an opportunity for venting, you may find it helpful to share your experiences with others who are dealing with pain issues. Ask your doctor or therapist for a local referral or get online and find one. If there is nothing local, there are also some great online pain support groups.

- Psychotherapy is helpful in learning how to cope with pain, and in resolving some of the underlying issues that have led to the development of chronic pain. A great deal of physical pain is caused by underlying residual trauma that manifests somatically (in the body). Again and again, I see clients who experienced cumulative or extreme trauma or abuse as children, coming in with unexplained pain issues. It's often not until we discuss when the pain started that the client makes the connection about her emotional experiences and her physical experiences. In particular, women who were sexually or physically abused as children may have numerous aches and pains, minor diseases or infections, or other medical conditions. None of this is your fault; all of it can be helped with psychotherapy.

Psychological and Emotional Pain

In addition to physical pain, there is mental, emotional, spiritual, and relational pain. All of it is inter-related. Although we often try to separate the body from the mind, we cannot truly separate the physical and the mental. Nonetheless, mental pain *is* a little different. Some people actually report a sensation that their brain hurts. They might say "Dr. Kubacky, I don't have a headache, but …. my brain HURTS!" I know that they're talking about an aspect of depression. This "brain pain" is associated with depression, chronic pain, and increased feelings of suicidality. As I said, depression hurts.

As a result of emotional injury, trauma, exposure to violence, child abuse, adult domestic violence, unhealthy relationships of all sorts, inadequate coping skills and feelings of overwhelm, you may have emotional pain. Some therapists refer to this as "psych-ache," which is a way of describing a pain in your psyche – a pain in your heart and soul. This may be an existential crisis in classical terms, or something that feels like an existential crisis – one of those eternal crises that we all face from time to time. Or it may be what my mentor terms a "spiritual crisis," one that only God/god can truly address. It may be the dominant force in your life, or something that just haunts you a bit here and there. This type of pain is best addressed through self-examination, creative work, and talk therapy.

When your experiences are heard and validated, you are taking a critical step in both owning those experiences and transforming them. You can make a choice to shift out of pain by acknowledging painful facts from the past. In addition to committing time and financial resources to therapy, you might need to take other actions. This could include developing a more extensive social support network, engaging in creative or spiritual practices, like reading, journaling, writing, and creating artwork, or practicing movement therapies, yoga, or taking long solitary walks.

Time is helpful. So is seeking help from a therapist. This process of unwinding from emotional pain can be a long one, with peaks and valleys. It may look like or even actually be depression for a while. It requires patience, and some courage, on the part of both the client and the therapist. Change is the result of an accumulation of small "snaps" that occur throughout the talk therapy process, the work that you do when you're away from the therapist, and what the therapist synthesizes and brings back into the therapy. It's a fabulously non-linear process. But I get it – sometimes that just feels ridiculously slow. And it might be, but the payoff is well worthwhile. In the meantime, please implement some of my quick tips for coping, found below.

Spiritual Pain

If the term "spiritual crisis" resonates for you on some level, you may be feeling a lack of a god/God/spirit/source in your life, feeling abandoned by god as you once knew him or her or it, feeling punished by god, or doubting the existence of god altogether. Perhaps you were an atheist, and now something about it doesn't feel quite right, but you don't know what other belief might feel good to you. Or you might have had negative experiences with religious institutions or spiritual leaders. If your parents shoved a particular brand of religion down your throat, you may have rejected it outright and now find yourself secretly yearning for it. Many people find that, as they grow older, have children, or go through challenging experiences of illness, they are more drawn to seek out the spiritual. For many, a sense of belonging and connection in the universe is derived from something they call a religion, or a form of spirituality. A lack of connection to others feels deeply painful.

Addressing an emotional or spiritual crisis is the same as addressing other forms of crisis. First, you need to know what the problem is. It may start with a vague sense of malaise, of not belonging, being off-kilter, out of sorts, or in constant need of realignment. You might notice that you're attracted to the sorts of semi-spiritual teachings you would have ignored before, like wondering a little bit more about that "deep" poem your yoga teacher read out loud at the end of class, trying to pull lessons from it.

If you can identify the problem, you can begin to know the solution. Sometimes, in these realms, it is lack of love we are feeling. That may be the love of others, or AN-other, but it may also be love of self. A crisis of self-love feels lonely, painful, and awkward, just the same as a crisis of romantic love. Part of coping, aside from the knowing what it is that is making you feel sorrowful, is knowing that you may have to live through and with some very uncomfortable feelings, often for quite a long time. I love the idea that you can snap your fingers and make it go away, but it's just not true. Our emotional states may be mercurial, but they tend to roll in waves. Know that it may take a while to pull yourself out of a slump.

Relational Pain

Human beings are wired to seek support, connection, and life with other human beings. When relationships are missing, impaired, or downright damaging, either in the present moment or in your past, you may have a lot of healing work to do. This work is what we do in psychotherapy. By seeking support and connection, you begin to experience trust and safety with your therapist, as you explore your relational wounds. As healing takes place in the therapist/patient relationship, you begin to become more able to connect with others, and more desirous of that connection.

A significant part of the relational pain of PCOS can be improved through seeking the support of other women with PCOS, participating in online activities, going to fundraisers and educational events, and offering your hard-earned wisdom to other women who are just starting their PCOS journeys. The power of the group is very healing.

Top 10 Quick Tips for Coping with Pain:

1. Get adequate sleep. See *Chapter 17: Improving Sleep.*
2. Identify good sources of social support and stay connected.
3. Identify a competent team of healthcare providers, even if you don't need a particular specialty now.
4. Learn what constitutes a proper dietary approach for YOU, and start implementing it.
5. Develop a competent, assertive, take-charge attitude about your PCOS.
6. Start exercising; it's good for your body and your mind.
7. Stick to your medication schedule.
8. Get mental health assistance if you have any suggestion of suffering from excess stress, anxiety, depression, mood swings or any suicidal thoughts at all.
9. Choose supplements with care, and experiment.
10. Identify key sources of stress and take steps to manage and reduce them.

Addressing the complexity of physical, mental, emotional, spiritual, and relational pain may seem daunting. However, it's necessary to enhancing your overall sense of well-being, improving your health, and reducing depression, anxiety, and other mood disorder symptoms. In the next chapter, we'll delve into one of the best tools for addressing all these issues: meditation.

CHAPTER 16
Developing a Meditation Practice

Among the most important skills I teach my clients is meditation. Almost everyone can meditate "successfully" with a little guidance, instruction, and practice. So, let's demystify meditation.

What IS Meditation?

Meditation is a state of "thoughtless awareness," in which the mind is quiet, yet alert. Technically speaking, it's not concentration or effort – although it certainly can feel like that, especially in the beginning! It is a practice of contemplation, thought, and reflection, performed in a focused way, with the intention of producing feelings of calm, relaxation, focus, and centeredness. For our purposes, I'm going to mix the terminology of guided visualization and meditation, because the goal is the same: emptying your mind to reduce your PCOS-related stress.

Meditation may be as simple as sitting still and trying to ignore distractions, and as complex as a lifetime dedicated to refinement of the practice. Either way, it is rewarding. There are probably about a dozen key forms of meditation, some of which have been practiced for thousands of years, while others are newer versions. But at their core, they all aim to reduce stress and produce a calm mental state by shutting down the hyperactive chit-chat in our brains. This chatter is often referred to as "Monkey Mind," which is exactly what it sounds like – all your thoughts jumbled up, bouncing around, and a little frenetic, like a bunch of little monkeys.

What Meditation is NOT

Meditation is part of many spiritual practices and communities, but meditation itself is neither religious nor spiritual. Meditation is not a cult. Meditation is not a substitute for mental health treatment; it complements it. Meditation is not one particular process, despite popular attempts to brand and sell meditation.

How Does Meditation Benefit PCOS?

There are numerous potential benefits of meditation for women with PCOS. These include:

Relaxation and stress reduction. It feels nice. And how much time do we spend actively pursuing things that feel pleasant for our minds and bodies? Meditation is a little daily gift to yourself. It can definitely feel a little stressful at first, when you're trying to figure out what to do and how to do it, but I promise, the calming benefits of meditation are both legendary and true. Time and practice will give you something very hard to find – that sense of being calm, focused, and centered solidly in yourself.

Improved quality of life. As you calm your mind, you are likely to see that your life is calming down too. Things that once stressed you out now have reduced effect. Your stress responses are slowed. You're less reactive. You respond better to people you once found aggravating. Your sense of humor returns or strengthens.

Improved psychoneuroimmunology. That's a big word naming the linkage of the immune system, the brain, chronic illness, stress, and mood. Psychological events and stressors affect the immune system negatively. In other words, stress makes you sick. More intriguingly, when stress occurs and cortisol is released, the body and brain produce some behavioral changes, in an effort to fight back while conserving resources.

These include changes in liver metabolism, reduced sexual activity, and increased anxiety, among other things.

Reduced healthcare costs. It's well-known that stress increases blood pressure, blood sugar, and anxiety/depression. The more proactively you manage your stress – meditation being a key tool – the less healthcare costs you're likely to have.

Improved fertility. Meditation decreases the monthly surge of luteinizing hormone, which triggers ovulation. Meditation also reduces insulin resistance and improves your overall sex hormone balance, both of which contribute to fertility.

Increased focus, memory, and sense of self-control. Since meditation is about focus, it makes sense that the practice itself will improve your ability to focus. More importantly, it strengthens the ability to *refocus*, which is very helpful since we are all constantly being pulled in different directions. By knowing how to clear out distractions quickly, a side effect is improved memory because you're actually paying attention better! Finally, knowing that you have this internal mastery gained by meditating regularly increases your sense of self-control and self-efficacy.

Decreased mental health/mood disorder symptoms. Major Depressive Disorder, Attention Deficit Disorder, and Generalized Anxiety Disorder are disorders that affect many women with PCOS, and meditation helps soothe you and increase your ability to cope with them. Multiple studies demonstrate both the restorative and reparative effects of meditation, particularly mindfulness meditation and Transcendental Meditation, on the brain. Increased focus and attention, decreased feelings of depression, and less anxiety are the remarkable benefits that you can obtain from consistently practicing meditation.

Improved sleep. The thing I hear repeatedly from the women in my practice is that they have sleep problems because their brains are still going in high gear at bedtime. There are many ways to work on improving sleep, as described in *Chapter 17*, but know that meditation will help you shut down your busy brain and get out of "spin cycle" or "monkey mind" much more quickly and easily. There are also specific pre-bedtime meditations that can help guide you into a deeper and more restful sleep in less time.

Decreased mood swings. Mood swings are a hallmark of PCOS, due to shifting and unreliable hormone levels. Mood swings are more common in women with bipolar disorder, menopause, peri-menopause, premenstrual syndrome, premenstrual dysphoric disorder, or clinical depression. Meditation has been shown to decrease mood swings present in all these conditions.

Other positive brain effects. Simply stated, the more you meditate, the more the good connections in your brain (the ones that enable empathy and the ability to quickly decrease fear) are strengthened, and the neural connections that lead to panic, anxiety, fear, and mistrust, or lack of empathy fade into the background. More technically, the lateral prefrontal cortex, which is the part of the brain that is the most logical and rational, is strengthened by meditation. This enhances your ability to override automatic responses generated by the medial prefrontal cortex, which processes information from an unhelpful (more selfish, less empathic) place. The amygdala, which is the part of your brain that senses danger and responds appropriately, is often overly active from the stress of daily living or from trauma in your past. Meditation tamps down those over activated fear sensors.

By now, I hope you're sold on the benefits of meditation, and just want to know how to get started and begin getting all those great benefits. The best way to get quick results is simply to start immediately, go with something simple, and release your focus on the outcome. Doing meditation once or even a few times doesn't have immediate results. Usually, it takes some time before you notice that you're experiencing the benefits I've described above.

Types of Meditation

There are many types of meditation. Here's a very brief overview of some of the most widely practiced, well-known, and popular forms of meditation.

Guided meditation is a popular way to meditate, and it's an easy way to get started without any special training. You can simply follow a guided meditation, led live by someone in a spiritual setting, yoga class, etc. But it's much easier to download one of the many apps that are now available, such as Insight, Calm, Simply Being, or Headspace. Pick one that sounds appealing (either by topic, teacher, or length), get comfortable, and hit play. You are meditating!

Mindfulness meditation is particularly popular now, and with good reason. Mindfulness, as described by Jon Kabat-Zinn, a famous teacher of meditation, is "paying attention in a particular way: on purpose, in the present moment, and nonjudgmentally." To start, sit comfortably, and begin noticing the moment. Notice what's going on in your body, your breath, and your mind. Judgments will come, and just let them roll right by. I often use the visual of a ticker tape machine running a constant stream of verbal "noise" inside your mind. Return your attention to the moment. Be kind to your mind and its tendency to wander. Keep cycling through this process. Go for a minute to 20 minutes. Congratulate yourself on increasing your mindfulness.

Guided visualization/progressive relaxation. Strictly speaking, these are not meditations, but from my perspective, they serve much the same purpose. Guided visualizations are similar to guided meditations, but often have more of a story or purpose to them, such as achieving deep relaxation. Similarly, progressive relaxation is what it sounds like – vocal and/or mental guidance through a body scan, head-to-toe or toe-to-head, where you clench and release your muscles sequentially. I usually do this over the course of about 20 minutes, and it's often relaxing enough to send you off to sleep easily. It can also be useful as a daily practice to lower stress on a consistent basis.

Mantra meditation. You may have heard the word "mantra," wondered if you needed one to start meditating and, if so, how you got one. The answer is no, you don't need one, but many people find it helpful, and this is a simple and common form of meditation. A mantra is simply a word or sound repeated to aid in your concentration while meditating. When your attention drifts – which it will – you bring your attention back to the mantra. Mantras may be assigned by spiritual leaders, Transcendental Meditation teachers (more on that below), or others, but you can simply pick a word or sound that resonates for you and use it as your focal point. Many people choose words like *peace, calm, harmony, joy, focus, love,* etc. You can change the mantra to suit your mood or need from day to day.

Transcendental Meditation (TM) is an evidence-based technique that has been found to be consistently effective, even for children, people with post-traumatic stress disorder, and those with Attention Deficit Disorder. It also has benefits for anxiety, cardiovascular health, depression, addiction, and Autism Spectrum Disorder. The downside is that it is only taught one-on-one, and it's expensive. There are TM communities around the world where you can practice with others, and there are numerous scholarships available for students who wish to learn the practice. I learned TM along with my entire family when I was 10 years old, and it is one of the forms of meditation I return to repeatedly, although not exclusively. In TM, a mantra is used to restore and maintain focus.

Moving meditation is a great alternative for children, people with ADD/ADHD, and others who literally cannot imagine themselves sitting still for even a few moments. There are formalized practices, such as Qigong or Tai Chi, which use rhythmic physical movements to focus the mind and body. There are also walking and dancing meditations that you can perform alone or with others. I often recommend walking meditation, which may be performed by deliberately slowly your movements to a snail's pace and focusing intensely on your environment. This may be done indoors, perhaps focusing on the pattern in a carpet. It's especially nice to do outdoors, because it enhances the healing connection with nature.

Breath focus meditation is what it sounds like. Instead of focusing on "nothing" or a mantra, you focus on your breath. When you get distracted, return to your breath.

If you're feeling more confused about where to start after reading these descriptions, sit quietly for a moment and see which one jumps out at you, seems most interesting, or resonates for you in some other way. There is a great deal of further instruction available online and in most communities, and if you don't like the first one you try, just try another form of meditation.

Starting Your Practice

Try a sample session. Let's keep this really simple to start. Set a timer for three minutes or five minutes (this helps, so you're not constantly opening your eyes to peek at the time). Sit in a chair or on a couch, feet on the floor, hands in your lap. Close your eyes. Focus on your breath. Get distracted. Refocus on your breath. As distracted thoughts continue to come through, quietly label them "thinking" or "thoughts" and let them go. Stop when the timer goes off. Congratulate yourself for having successfully meditated!

Posture, props/equipment, and setting. The truth is, you need nothing more than a place to sit and your good intentions, but many people find it helpful to set the mood by creating an environment that supports contemplative behavior. As you develop skills, you will be able to meditate with a crying baby, on an airplane, or in a noisy office setting too.

Choose a quiet spot. This might mean waking up a few minutes early, so you have the house to yourself, stepping out to your yard and closing the door, or locking yourself in the spare bedroom. If you're meditating during the day when you're at work or out and about, a spare office, a park or courtyard, or even your parked car are suitable locations.

Candles/incense. If you like the idea of lighting a candle or incense to start your practice and add some atmosphere, go for it. If you're allergic, stick with unscented candles. And of course, don't forget to extinguish them when you're finished, or your equilibrium may soon be disrupted by a fire crisis.

Music. Although many guided meditations include some instrumental music in the background, it's not necessary, and may even be a distraction. Try it and see how you respond. An advanced technique is using a Tibetan "singing bowl" to begin and end your session. These bowls have a lovely tone and are very beautiful.

Cushions used for meditation and yoga are called Zafus, which translates to "sit cushion." They are typically round, small, and very firm, just enough to prop you up and support a correct seated posture. If you end up wanting to formalize your practice a little more, adding some of these props can be nice. There are some very beautiful Zafus.

Phone applications (Apps) and online audios or videos demonstrating or leading you in meditation are also useful. There are literally thousands of them. Some are free, some require a fee. Sample a good handful to see what suits you and if you use something like the Insight App, there are new offerings every day. The body likes routine, but the brain thrives on novelty, so don't worry if you get bored easily and want to switch it up.

Tips and Troubleshooting

Establish a regular practice. Like exercise, I find that meditating first thing in the morning is one of the best ways to make sure that it happens. Otherwise, you get distracted and it just seems to never happen. Meditation, while relaxing, is also just enough of a stimulant to bring you into the day more fully. And for those of us who are not morning people, it tends to ease the transition from cranky early morning to a more pleasant and engaging public persona.

Commit mentally and emotionally to just five minutes a day. If that's too much, start with one minute or even 30 seconds a day. ANY meditation is more beneficial than none, and like anything else, as you gain comfort with the practice, you will be able to extend it. The ultimate goal is 20 minutes per day (twice a day if time permits). Like walking, take the approach of doing five minutes for a couple of weeks. Then increase to 10 minutes for a week or two, and so on, until you have reached 20 minutes per day. As you get into the habit of the practice, you may even find yourself craving the meditation time, and wanting to lengthen it naturally, without having to force it.

Be patient. Be kind to yourself. Like any skill, meditation takes some time to learn. With consistency, your ability or tolerance builds up. Seek out some other people who meditate and talk to them for support.

Know that meditation is about letting go/surrendering. Sometimes, I think the sense of overwhelm about meditation, the worry and the wonder about it, is actually a gift. If you allow yourself to surrender to the mystery of it, stop judging, and let it unfold, it's a great metaphor for the life that we cannot control. And it's a reminder that letting go often ends up feeling better than fighting, if you do it with consciousness.

Meditate with others. You can do this by joining a meditation group at a local yoga studio or Buddhist temple, or by going on a retreat that includes meditation. You can also take advantage of the collective energy to be found on Apps like Insight, which let you know how many people meditated with you. It can be a positive reinforcement to have professional or guided instruction, and to feel the "vibes" of the other meditators. I always leave such experiences feeling energized.

Let go of perfectionism and competitiveness. If you've got any latent tendencies towards perfectionism or competitiveness, they will surely arise in meditation, just as they do everywhere else. Meditation is the antithesis of these traits. You cannot win, and you cannot be perfect when you do it. And that is quite freeing and relaxing!

Take advantage of your resources. A number of meditation resources are listed in the Resources section at the back of this book, including some of my favorite Apps and websites that support meditation. I also regularly try out new things and talk about them on the PCOS Wellness website and blogs, and in the PCOS Psychology Facebook group, which I invite you to join today, if you haven't already.

Meditation is an ancient practice with powerful implications for modern living, especially for women with PCOS. The benefits may include reduced insulin resistance and blood pressure, enhanced fertility, sleep improvements, and an overall sense of calm. It's free and easy to start, and absolutely possible to carve out five minutes in your day to give this gift to yourself. The methods above will make it even easier.

CHAPTER 17
Improving Sleep

There are only two things you should be doing in bed, sleeping and having sex. This chapter is all about getting high-quality sleep. When you engage in other activities in bed such as reading, playing games, watching TV, or eating, your brain learns to associate the bed and the bedroom with waking, alertness, and engagement - all of which are contrary to the goal of sleep. Multi-tasking, electric lights, electronic devices, and non-stop schedules are all contributors to sleep issues.

Two-thirds of people have occasional sleep problems, and one-quarter have chronic sleep problems. And consistent with the theme that PCOS causes more problems than average, of course women with PCOS tend to have more sleep problems. We really do need at least eight hours per night to ensure optimal functioning. Seven is a bare minimum and frankly, nine is optimal. If you're not getting adequate restorative sleep, you won't be energetic and ready to get out there and engage in the world, which may lead to some more serious health and social consequences.

The serious fallout of chronic sleep deprivation or disruption shows up in a variety of ways. Your immune system is negatively affected by lack of sleep, leaving you more vulnerable to infection and other stress-related illnesses. Poor sleep can cause or contribute to weight gain. It may also be a symptom or cause of heart disease, particularly if you have undetected or untreated sleep apnea, which I'll talk about in more detail. Occasional insomnia is annoying, but it won't really harm you. Extended insomnia, however, can cause or contribute to depression. It can make people with anxiety disorders more anxious as well. You may literally be wearing out your body faster than you should be. Let's look at what the problems are, and then we'll explore solutions.

Types of Sleep Disorders

In addition to the best-known sleep disorder, **insomnia** (where you have difficulty falling asleep, staying asleep, or getting good quality sleep for more than a month), there are a number of other sleep disorders, including:

Hypersomnia – excessive sleepiness for at least a month. It often occurs in conjunction with obstructive sleep apnea and/or obesity. Hypersomnia is a symptom of depression as well.

Nightmare disorder/night terrors. If you have recurrent nightmares or other frightening dreams that cause you to wake up in a state of stress, you may develop cumulative fatigue that is actually a sleep disorder.

Breathing-related sleep disorders. You might have excessive daytime sleepiness or fatigue because of **Obstructive Sleep Apnea**. Symptoms include loud snoring, breathing pauses that disrupt sleep, sleep that doesn't refresh, and waking with a headache in the morning. There is a much higher occurrence of sleep apnea among women with PCOS, and sleep apnea can contribute to the development or exacerbation of heart disease and diabetes, among other issues. It's very important to see a pulmonologist or other sleep specialist for further assessment if you have these symptoms. Severe untreated sleep apnea may result in premature death.

Parasomnias are unusual movement-related behavior during sleep, often sleepwalking, getting up to eat while asleep (reported with some medications as well), or sometimes having sex during sleep without being aware of it. Restless leg syndrome, while not a psychological disorder, is a related medical disorder that can cause sleep disruption.

Dyssomnias. A broad term covering problems falling asleep, staying asleep, or sleeping too much – any time your amount, quality or sleep timing is off, it's called a dyssomnia. The more commonly used term insomnia will tell any expert what they need to know though.

Narcolepsy. Described as "repeated irresistible attacks of refreshing sleep" coupled with some other symptoms. Although rare, it can be very dangerous (say, when driving, caring for a child, in a pool, etc.) because of its surprise nature.

Circadian rhythm sleep disorder. This form of insomnia most often occurs as a result of jet lag, shift work, or after having a significant disruption to your sleep schedule, like pulling an all-nighter before a big exam. Basically, your body is just so OFF, it can't or won't get to sleep.

Substance-induced sleep disorders. These result from the use of substances, or recent discontinuation of substances, causing sleep disruptions. For example, if you've been relying on marijuana to help you sleep, stopping smoking it may result in insomnia. This can include alcohol, prescription medications, and illicit drugs.

Sleep disorders related to a general medical condition. This occurs when your sleep disorder comes about as a result, or side effect, of a medical condition. Several chronic diseases disrupt sleep. These include kidney disease, diabetes and pre-diabetes (because of irregularities in blood sugars, as well as the frequent need to get up to urinate during the night), cardiovascular disease, thyroid disease, heartburn, gastrointestinal disorders like Crohn's disease, neurological diseases, and pain disorders. Many medications used to treat medical conditions may also disrupt sleep. Statins, beta-blockers, and SSRIs (antidepressants) are common culprits.

If you have any of these symptoms, behaviors, or concerns, it's important to get assessed by the appropriate medical professional, or a team of professionals. Your doctor could be the first stop and would be the person who would refer you for an overnight sleep study at a sleep lab if sleep apnea is suspected. Your therapist can also assess for sleep issues, provide behavioral treatments and lifestyle modifications, and make appropriate medical referrals. If you have complex or long-standing sleep issues, you might need to add a medical sleep specialist, typically a pulmonologist, or a behavioral sleep specialist, like a psychologist who specializes in sleep disorders.

Complications of Sleep Disorders

To expand upon what I listed above, the effects of sleep problems are system-wide and often dire. It's not just about being tired. Your immune system is negatively affected by lack of sleep. When you already have a chronic illness such as PCOS, you are more vulnerable to infectious diseases anyway. The body is chronically taxed and has less resources available to fight off other germs, bacteria, and viruses. If you have other related conditions, such as diabetes, you have an even greater vulnerability to infection.

Poor sleep can cause or contribute to weight gain. This is related both to the effects of cortisol (your body is always in panic mode and sending out surges of cortisol) as well as being so tired from lack of sleep that you a) don't get up early enough to exercise or can't last late enough in the day to do it; b) don't exercise at all, regardless of time of day; or c) eat more, typically carbohydrates, in an effort to produce serotonin, get the energy that comes from a glucose surge, and make yourself feel better. If you're thinking "wow, that sounds like a vicious circle," you are correct – and it is very, very common for women with PCOS.

Numerous studies have linked insomnia, sleep apnea, and other sleep disorders with an increased risk of heart disease. Since PCOS already gives you an increased risk of heart disease, I say, why add fuel to the fire?

Insomnia is insidious in that it can cause or exacerbate depression. Chronic insomnia can actually cause a full-blown major depressive episode, which is much harder to treat than a mild depressive episode. It also takes longer. If you're already dealing with depression, it can make it worse, or make it harder to get rid of. If you have bipolar disorder, insomnia can be extra dangerous, as it can trigger manic or hypomanic episodes.

Insomnia can also make you really grumpy, which has negative effects on your relationships, your work life, and your family life. When you're irritable, people don't like to be around you, and you don't like to be around them. This may lead to isolation –yet another symptom of depression.

Taking Action to Improve Your Sleep

Are you now convinced that you've got to do something about your sleep? The rest of this chapter is about how to address sleep problems on your own. *If you suspect that you have sleep apnea, don't just try the DIY approaches first; call a doctor immediately to schedule a medical assessment.* I'm convinced that when you see how easily you can improve your sleep, and how much better you feel when your sleep is good, you will want to keep up with these changes. This includes information about what you're consuming, correcting or enhancing the sleep environment, supplements you can use, and behaviors you can change to improve your sleep.

Substances Affecting Sleep: The Bad

Caffeine. You don't need a doctor to tell you to drink less coffee and see if it helps you sleep, but I'm going to do that anyway! The bottom line is, caffeine negatively affects sleep. The surprise, however is that a) you may be more sensitive to it than you realize; b) you may be consuming far more than you realize; c) you might need to stop consuming caffeine as early as noon (or even – ack! – altogether!) to improve your sleep patterns. Many people become more sensitive to caffeine as they age, so what was once okay, like a quick latte at 4:00 p.m. when you're slumping at work, may now be the direct cause of your insomnia. Move the dial back by two hours on the last dose of caffeine and see how it goes. If that's not enough, try cutting yourself off at noon. Don't forget to check the caffeine content of your favorite beverages; caffeine hides in light-colored sodas, chocolate, diet cola, green tea, and energy drinks. Extremely sensitive individuals may even be affected by coffee-flavored ice cream, candies, or desserts.

Sugar is a stimulant. Sugar gives you a buzz, and sugar makes you crash. It wreaks havoc on your blood chemistry and hormonal balance and will disrupt sleep as surely as caffeine. So, if you're in the habit of dessert after dinner, drinking several sweetened coffees or sugar-sweetened sodas or juices during the day, or snacking on candy, you may want to experiment with eliminating the sugar, or at least stopping it after midday. That will also help with improving your diet, if sugar is generally a problem for you. By restricting or eliminating sugar, you will be contributing to improved hormonal balance.

Alcohol. It may seem like a glass of alcohol before bed makes you sleepy, but at 2:00 a.m., the buzz that sedated you in the first place is going to wear off, and you'll probably wake up and have difficulty falling back asleep. Alcohol itself contains no sugar, but the mixers are usually loaded with sugar. The last thing a woman with PCOS needs is more sugar in her system. That doesn't mean you shouldn't drink, but make it worthwhile and not a nightly thing.

Substances Affecting Sleep: The Good

Tryptophan. It's in turkey, milk, and other forms of dairy. A little turkey breast before you turn in may be something that gets you to sleep through the night. Likewise, a glass of milk or some yogurt may help you sleep. Try it for a few nights and see if you notice an improvement.

Calcium. Of course, it's found in dairy products, kale, and sardines (among other calcium-rich foods), but a calcium supplement, if appropriate for you, taken before bed can also help improve sleep.

Magnesium. Beans, nuts, whole-grain foods, and dark leafy greens are all good sources of magnesium. These are also good healthy foods in general. Women with PCOS are almost universally deficient in magnesium, which contributes not only to sleep problems, but also to depression and gastrointestinal problems. If you're not getting enough in your diet, over-the-counter magnesium supplements may be helpful. Just be mindful that too much can cause diarrhea, as it's a systemic relaxant. Magnesium is absorbed through the skin, so bathing in Epsom salts can be helpful, as can topical magnesium sprays. In short, if you're not sleeping well or have even progressed to full-blown insomnia, try these dietary suggestions before you try over-the-counter or prescription sleep medication. The power to improve your sleep quantity and quality may well lie in what you put in your body.

Behaviors That Improve Sleep

In addition to paying attention to what you eat and drink, there are many behavioral modifications that are helpful for improving your sleep. Try the following:

- Establish a regular, relaxing bedtime routine. Relaxing rituals prior to bedtime may include a warm bath or shower, washing your face, using aromatherapy, reading, or listening to soothing music.
- Sleep in a room that is quiet and comfortable. If there are noises you can't control, consider investing in an inexpensive white noise machine that masks annoying sounds with more soothing sounds.
- Make sure the temperature in your bedroom is comfortable. Low temperatures (under 70F) are often recommended, but a slightly warm room may make you feel sleepier. Experiment until you find what works for you. You may need to do a little semi-scientific experimentation with this, adjusting one element per night until you get it right – blanket versus down comforter, 70 degrees versus 68 degrees, pants on versus pants off, etc., so be patient. Like any other experiment, go for the easiest elements first.
- Sleep in darkness. Even the slightest light leaks can disrupt your sleep, so make sure your room is as dark as possible. Buy some inexpensive blackout shades or curtains if necessary. And, if you need to get up in the middle of the night to go to the bathroom, don't turn any lights on.
- Sleep on a comfortable mattress and pillows and make sure your linens are comfortable as well (nothing itchy, scratchy, or rough).
- Finish eating at least two to three hours before your regular bedtime.
- Snack right. Nighttime low blood sugar is a frequent cause of waking. Avoid sugars before bed, which will peak and then fall rapidly. Instead, have a high-protein snack, which provides

the L-tryptophan necessary for production of melatonin and serotonin. Also, avoid foods you may be sensitive to, such as wheat or dairy, which may cause nausea, gas, or congestion.

- Avoid smoking within two hours of bedtime. Really, you should never smoke, but if you must indulge, remember that nicotine is a stimulant that will keep you awake.

- Exercise regularly. As with eating, finish at least two to three hours before bedtime. Even better, do it in the morning. Thirty minutes per day, every day, helps ensure that you can fall asleep easily. Exercising closer to bedtime may cause disruptions in your sleep pattern because you're overly activated by the exercise. The exception would be practicing a brief yoga sequence especially designed to encourage sleep.

- Skip the naps, as enticing as they may be, so that you are actually tired enough to sleep at night. If you're using regular naps to fill a sleep deficit, you are encouraging the problematic nighttime sleep issues.

- Never work in bed. You will associate bed with work and alertness, which is counterproductive to sleep. Turn the computer off, put the phone away, and finish electronic games at least two hours before your scheduled bedtime. This allows your brain to slow down from its usual intense processing and problem-solving mode. And keep your work materials and computer in another room; their mere presence can cause distress and distraction.

- No watching TV in bed. Television offers too much stimulation, even when it's mind-numbingly bad TV.

- Plan for a morning brain dump to start your day off right. This requires you to keep an empty journal or notebook by your bed. As soon as you wake up, and the thoughts about all the things you have to do come flooding in, start writing. Write for 20 minutes or three pages, whichever comes first. Don't worry about punctuation, spelling, grammar, or continuity of thought. Just spew.

- Go to bed at the same time every night and get up at the same time every morning. This helps your body acclimate to the routine of consistent sleep. This means weekends too. It may feel hard to resist sleeping in at first, but you will become more comfortable physically if you keep things consistent.

- Once you've turned the lights off, give yourself 20 minutes to get to sleep. If you don't fall asleep, get up and go do something relatively mindless for an hour, and try again. Repeat until you eventually fall asleep. Do not stay in bed "resting" and staring at the ceiling for hours; this merely teaches your brain that bed is a place for being awake. You will not derive any functional benefit from this type of rest.

- Limit your use of over-the-counter sleep aids like Benadryl, Tylenol PM, Advil PM, or Unisom; they can be addictive, ineffective, or cause a rebound effect (worse insomnia) when you stop them.

- Get evaluated for sleep apnea if you have any of the following symptoms: waking up feeling groggy or unrested, snoring, waking with a start in the middle of the night with your heart racing and/or feeling fearful, insulin resistance (abdominal fat), and/or family history of sleep apnea or crib death. The older you get, the more likely you are to have sleep apnea, and women with PCOS have it with an alarming degree of frequency.

- If you have (or suspect you have) allergies, get them diagnosed and treated so you can breathe more easily. This may include allergy shots, eliminating problematic substances, encasing your bedding to protect against dust and dust mites, running a special air filter, using an inhaler, nasal washing, or prescription medication. Many allergy medications that used to be available only by prescription are now available over-the-counter. These may be helpful as well.

- Along with allergies, many women with PCOS also have asthma. Even mild asthma can interfere significantly with nighttime breathing and restorative sleep. An allergist can treat asthma along with allergies.

- Tilt the bed up 4-6" to reduce/eliminate a condition called silent reflux (gastrointestinal distress, acid secretion), which is very common in overweight people, and may interfere with sleep. If you find that helpful, great, but don't skip getting a proper evaluation and treatment from a gastroenterologist.

- Get evaluated for depression. Any licensed psychotherapist can assess you for depression and make appropriate treatment recommendations. This may include a suggestion to try antidepressants, which can help with sleep.

- Get your hormones checked. As a woman with PCOS, you've probably already done this, but, if you haven't, get your hormones checked by your gynecologist or natural health practitioner. You may be experiencing sleep disruption related to peri-menopause or menopause.

- Try melatonin. For many people, occasional use of melatonin is enough to help them restore their normal sleep cycles. It is available over the counter, but of course, check with your doctor first to see if it's appropriate for you. The proper dose is ½ mg (500 mcg) a few hours before bedtime if your problem is falling asleep, and/or ½ mg (500 mcg) at bedtime if you have a problem with waking in the middle of the night.

- Consider using other natural sleep aids such as 5-HTP, GABA, or L-theanine. Some of these supplements are powerfully effective in promoting good quality sleep. They are described more fully in *Chapter 11: Selective Supplementation and Other Tools.*

- Try herbs such as chamomile, valerian root, kava kava, lemon balm, and hops. Chamomile tea is a pleasant and easy pre-bed prescription.

- Keep a sleep log, noting times, place, quality of sleep, what you ate, etc. You might be surprised at the patterns that are revealed. Share this information with your therapist and your doctor; it can be very helpful in treating your sleep problem.

- Add a defined period of relaxation to your night time routine. Watch some mindless television, read fashion magazines or catalogs, doodle in a notebook, or stare vacantly into space for a while before bed. Your body will learn to respond in a positively Pavlovian way when your start your nightly ritual.

- Get a prescription for sleeping pills, if needed, and use them for a limited time, strictly according to doctor's orders. I've often seen a one-week course of prescription sleep medication, followed by a week of every other night use, serve as a systemic re-set. Ambien, Rozerem, and Lunesta are common brands. Long-term use of prescription sleep aids is rarely recommended and has been correlated with higher rates of premature death. You want to get at the root of the problem and use the appropriate remedies, whether they are psychological or medical in nature.

Getting adequate, high-quality, restorative sleep is critical to your health and well-being. It is especially important if you have anxiety, depression, or other psychological issues. Don't ignore symptoms of sleep apnea, depression, or gastrointestinal disease. There are many simple things you can try yourself to improve sleep quality and quantity. The payoff in improving your health will be immeasurable. Combined with exercise (our next topic), you've got a power-packed, life-improvement plan.

CHAPTER 18
Exercising for Health

B y now, you've probably been told "you need to exercise more" about a million times. That may or may not be true, depending upon your particular body, circumstances, and other health conditions. It might actually be that you need to exercise less! What is true, however, is that exercise will help almost anyone improve mental health.

Exercise is recommended so frequently for women with PCOS because it has a phenomenal number of benefits, such as:

Weight control. This is probably the number one reason exercise is recommended – basically, anything to get the weight down. Exercise does help with weight reduction (because that's what is meant by weight "control"), but not as much as you would think. It's perhaps 20% of the equation. There's an assumption that food choices are the other 80%, but stress management and inflammation management are also key factors in weight management when you have PCOS.

Increased strength. Muscle takes less space than fat (so you can look smaller, even if you weigh the same), and it burns more calories, even when at rest. And hey, who doesn't want "free" calorie burns? One of the gifts we have as women with PCOS is that we build muscle more easily than other women.

Fat loss. The holy grail of almost all PCOS treatment plans is the ever-elusive weight reduction/fat loss. When you exercise, you do burn calories, which can lead to fat loss. This is good because too much fat is bad for your organs, your overall functioning, and usually your self-esteem.

Reduced risk of cardiovascular disease. This one's a biggie for those of us with PCOS, especially as we get older. We have significantly higher rates of cardiovascular disease than the average woman. One way to keep heart disease at bay is to engage in regular exercise that strengthens your cardiovascular system. A bonus is that you will feel more energized when your brain is well oxygenated by exercise, and likely less depressed as well.

Decreased insulin resistance and lower risk of type 2 diabetes. Insulin resistance is tied to most, if not all, PCOS symptoms. Insulin resistance is never (as far as I know) a good thing. Most of us have it. When you exercise, your body burns glycogen, which is a form of glucose (sugar) that is stored in your muscles. When you finish with your exercise, drawing glucose from the bloodstream replenishes the glycogen stores in the muscles. The result is lower blood sugars. The more glycogen you burn, the better your insulin sensitivity becomes. This doesn't mean that you should exercise excessively, but you do need to exercise consistently to maintain the benefits.

Reduced blood pressure. By regularly stressing your heart, you develop increased cardiovascular strength, which means that your heart doesn't have to work as hard to pump blood throughout your body. The force on your arteries decreases, which results in a lower blood pressure number. This is a pretty consistent positive effect of exercise. If you're in the danger zone for possible/probable/developing high blood pressure, implementing an exercise program may take you right back down to normal. New guidelines mean that any blood pressure reading higher than 130/80 will be classified as high blood pressure, with a possible recommendation for medication to lower it. Slightly lower numbers may be even better.

Reduced risk of breast cancer. Breast cancer has been linked to obesity, especially after menopause. Regular exercise can decrease this risk.

Stronger bones and muscles. Resistance exercise (working out with weights, as opposed to doing cardiovascular exercise) strengthens both your bones and your muscles. Stronger muscles make life easier. I really like functional fitness training, which simulates the movements you need to do to engage in all your daily life activities. It also emphasizes core strength. Functional fitness helps directly with things like lifting, squatting, bending, picking up heavy or awkward stuff, and moving in other practical ways. Also of great importance to women is building bone mass, so that you don't end up with osteopenia or osteoporosis, two very painful and dangerous degenerative bone conditions that commonly afflict older women.

Improved balance. By engaging in exercise that develops strength and requires coordinated movement, you enhance your proprioception (sensing your relative position in space, and strength), balance, and ability to recover from accidents or potential injuries (a slip and fall, a misstep, etc.). It also helps you move more gracefully when you're not exercising.

Increased flexibility. Flexibility enables you to move with ease and function better in your daily life. It saddens me to see people who haven't continuously worked on their flexibility lose most of it as they age. If you want to maintain your health and independence for as long as possible, flexibility is key.

Better mental health and mood. This is an amazing benefit of exercise. When you exercise, you not only release the feel-good chemicals in the brain, but you also reduce immune system factors that can worsen depression. The feel-good chemicals are found in the neurotransmitters, endorphins, and endocannabinoids (a system of retrograde neurotransmitters that binds with cannabinoids naturally occurring in your system) that are often deregulated in people with depression or other mood disorders. Additionally, it can serve as a distraction from your worries or negative thinking, increase social interactions, and help you improve your confidence in your body and your ability to develop new skills. Some forms of exercise serve as a sort of moving meditation, which is an added layer of benefit. By reducing insulin resistance (and thus, inflammation), you may also be staving off one of the worst brain illnesses, Alzheimer's Disease.

Starting an Exercise Routine

If you're wondering what kind of exercise is best for mental health conditions, my answer is always "the exercise that you're willing to do regularly." If you force yourself to do exercise that you hate, you're probably going to lose your commitment and enthusiasm quickly, may be more likely to get injured, will probably feel bored and resentful, and if you give up quickly, you can add feelings of shame and guilt for having "failed." Let's short-circuit that by choosing something you at least like and find manageable. I'm not asking you to love it, because I'm realistic. If you end up loving it, that's fabulous. Liking and tolerating is good enough for now though.

That being said, I think it's a really good idea to start out slowly and gently. And of course, with the approval of your doctor. The number one exercise I recommend is walking. I'm also a big fan of yoga, Pilates, swimming, and strength training. I don't personally like running, but I'm including it here because a lot of people with anxiety find a combination of running and yoga to be ideal for symptom management. Anything that gets you up off the couch and moving around counts as movement though, including yard work, active child care, housekeeping, sightseeing, shopping, dancing, and even sex. Although some of these things are not "exercise" per se, the more active you are, the better you are likely to feel, physically and mentally. The specific benefits of some different types of exercise include:

Walking

- Lose weight/maintain healthy weight.
- Manage high blood pressure, heart disease, pre-diabetes, and type 2 diabetes.
- Improve bone and muscle strength.
- Improve mood.
- Improve balance and coordination.
- Reduce stress.

- Increase your Vitamin D levels, if done outside.
- Increase the concentration of norepinephrine, which modulates the brain's response to stress.

That is a whole lot of benefit for something as simple as walking, which we do every single day. The idea of starting may still sound daunting though, so let me tell you how I started a walking program that resulted in the loss of 70 pounds 20 years ago. I had not been exercising at all, so I literally started with five minutes a day. FIVE MINUTES! You can do it, I'm positive. Do that five minutes a day, every single day, for two weeks. Increase your time to 10 minutes a day. Walk 10 minutes a day for two weeks. Then increase it to 15 minutes a day for two weeks. Don't worry about how long it's going to take to get to some magical desirable length of time, whether you need to acquire a Fitbit, or anything else. If your doctor says it's okay, it's okay.

You need nothing more than comfortable shoes. At the beginning, you don't even need athletic shoes. Later, as you increase your endurance and the length of time that you're walking, you can get the fancy trackers, stylish shoes, and sun protective garb. I worked my way up to 75 minutes a day in about six months by following this plan. Along the way, I picked up a workout buddy at my office, and we walked and talked together through every lunch hour, and then ate lunch at our desks while doing some paperwork.

Like I said, I ended up losing 70 pounds in the space of about a year, and I built a sustainable habit that can be practiced almost anywhere. I also learned that walking is uniquely useful for people with insulin resistance, which reinforced that this was a good choice.

Yoga

This has been shown to have an astonishing number of benefits for women with PCOS, including stress reduction, improved blood test markers such as cholesterol, reduced adrenal and cortisol (the stress hormone) levels, decreased inflammation, and improved menstrual regularity, among others. Unless you have a contraindication like a significant back or neck injury, I recommend yoga for everyone with PCOS. Further benefits that can be experienced by everyone who practices yoga, not just women with PCOS, include:

- Increased flexibility which helps prevent injury, as described above.
- Increased strength and muscular tone. A lot of people think of yoga as being about flexibility and balance, which it is, but it's also considered a strength exercise, which makes it an even better choice.
- Cardiovascular health/improved breathing. Depending upon the style of yoga you choose to practice, some of the sequences can move fairly quickly, which may result in cardiovascular benefit.
- Improved circulation. Much of yoga is designed to increase circulation, with the goal of positively affecting the brain, thyroid, pelvic organs, and heart.
- Balancing metabolism. Certain yoga poses stimulate your organs, including your thyroid. I think that the reputed thyroid and other metabolic benefits probably require more frequent and focused yoga than most of us are likely to practice, but still, it can't hurt.
- Stress/anxiety reduction. People with anxiety tend to find yoga particularly helpful. It lowers blood pressure and produces feelings of calm, restfulness, and being centered. The breathing practices and reminders to stay present in the moment help reduce anxiety both temporarily and longer term.
- Weight reduction may result from the increased calories burned when you engage in yoga.
- Increased alertness/decreased tension. Yoga contains many restful and restorative poses, which will help you gain or regain focus and clarity, while simultaneously decreasing stress and tension.
- Learn to stay present in the moment.
- Help reduce anxiety, both temporarily and longer term.

- Help manage chronic pain. Chronic pain causes a decrease in brain matter (incredible, huh?), and yoga counteracts that by increasing grey matter and improving neuroplasticity. There are many adaptive yoga programs available, often combined with meditation, guided visualization, and other approaches that are helpful for managing pain.
- Neurotransmitter activity increases with consistent yoga practice. In particular, it boosts GABA, one of the calming neurotransmitters. Just one hour of yoga, a common class length, boosts GABA by 27%. This is why doing a little pre-bedtime yoga may be helpful. GABA tells your brain to "shut up and calm down."
- It reduces fatigue. By improving circulation, focusing on the present moment, and eliminating outside stressors while moving rhythmically, the exercises or postures in yoga can leave you feel simultaneously energized and relaxed.
- Decreases inflammation. Yoga reduces levels of stress hormones that promote inflammation. It also reduces some of the pro-inflammatory molecules in the body, including cytokines, which contribute to severe pain.
- Increases acceptance. Yoga encourages you to honor the state of your body and mind in the moment, accept that it will be different from day to day, and practice to practice. Sometimes, you're flexible and graceful, and other times, every pose seems awkward and difficult. Literally, "go with the flow" is the mantra of yoga. Yoga is also something that can be done by virtually anyone, regardless of age, gender, ability, disability, and certainly regardless of weight. Seeing many bodies at all different skill levels and states of imperfection is a great way to increase acceptance of your own body.

Are you sold on yoga by now? If so, great. You can start to practice in several ways. Ideally, go to a few beginner's classes or private lessons at the gym or a yoga studio so you can get quality instruction from a certified and experienced instructor. They will have mats and props for you to use while you figure out what you like. There are free community classes at most yoga studios, and an astonishing number of low-cost introductory packages available on Groupon, Living Social, etc. Look for a teacher who is supportive, gentle, and provides good corrective direction so that you are safe when practicing. If that's not possible, there are also a lot of instructors who post videos on YouTube. I really like *Yoga With Adriene*. She has a gentle, positive, and encouraging approach to teaching. Check for the most experienced ones, make sure you don't do anything too uncomfortable, and go slowly and carefully, and you can learn at home.

When you get a little more comfortable and advanced in your yoga practice, you can use your skills while standing or sitting, as a breathing practice in the car, or even in the office if you have space with a clean enough floor. I also like to practice outside, either at the beach or in my backyard, on the grass, when weather and time permit. It's fun to practice with a partner as well.

Pilates

This is another one of my favorite physical activities. It's one of the safest forms of exercise/strength training you can do and gives you long, lean, elegant muscles. Additional benefits of Pilates include:

- Improved flexibility from the coordinated movements.
- Equalizing/balancing strength and flexibility on both sides of the body – everything in Pilates is done symmetrically, so you literally almost can't overdevelop or underwork any one part.
- Long, lean muscles. Did I mention the long, lean muscles? Google some pictures of Pilates instructors and you'll see what I mean. Even if you've got fat over those muscles, your whole body will look better.
- Enhanced core strength (abdominals, lower back, hips and buttocks). This is all about strengthening the core, but it's not all about doing hundreds of crunches.

- Better posture is a natural outcome of a stronger core and more evenly developed musculature. Pilates focuses a lot of attention on developing a strong, straight back and proper alignment.
- Injury rehabilitation/prevention. Pilates was originally developed as a physical therapy/injury recovery method for dancers, but it is helpful for everyone.
- Improved concentration – it requires focus on your breath, as well as the physical movements.
- Pilates teachers will identify specific muscles, and focus on refined and precise technique, which increases body awareness.
- Stress reduction comes through focus, concentration, and being "just Zen enough" as you practice.
- Improved cardiovascular health/breathing technique, as described above, which can also be enhanced if you participate in jumpboard classes, which are true cardio. The jumpboard is a device that attaches to the front of the Pilates Reformer machine, turning it into a horizontal jumping device.

There are two ways to do Pilates. One of them involves machines, boxes, and other props called the Reformer, the Tower, etc. These machines are fairly expensive and take up a lot of space, so you will need to go to a gym or other training facility and work with a certified Pilates teacher. You will use props such as rings, blocks, and balls. Classes are typically a little less than an hour. They're not cheap, but definitely more affordable than taking private lessons, which is also an option (and, like yoga, the optimal way to start so you can get comfortable with the equipment and terminology before jumping into a group class). Because of this, Pilates Reformer classes are usually small – about five or six machines – although I've seen studios with as many as a dozen in a room.

The other way to begin practicing Pilates also gives a very high level of benefit, but is less expensive and more accessible, because it doesn't require the use of machines. This is called Pilates mat work, and involves many of the same movements, but they are performed standing, sitting, or on the floor. You may use props such as hand weights or balls. Pilates mat classes are often offered by the same studios that have the machines, but for a much lower fee. They may also be offered at your local gym for free, as part of your monthly membership fee. Like yoga, you will find many classes online as well. Videos online are another option, once you've learned the basics in a class, so you can stay safe.

Swimming and Aqua Jogging

Both swimming and a related activity, aqua jogging, are often recommended for overweight people, people with chronic pain, or people with injuries. You undoubtedly already know what swimming is, but you may not be familiar with aqua jogging. Aqua jogging requires use of a water-resistant flotation belt, which come in sizes to fit even very large waists. Like swimming, aqua jogging is performed in a swimming pool. Swimming can be a very relaxing activity, as well as being a great cardiovascular activity. Aqua jogging is what it sounds like: jogging or running in the water. It can be a sociable activity if performed in a group. It's good for developing stamina and core muscles, as well as providing a surprisingly good workout, especially when paired with resistance training involving water barbells and other equipment. If you don't know how to swim yet, most YMCAs and public recreational programs offer low-cost options for adult learners. And you do not need to know how to swim to do aqua jogging! You can practice your skills on vacation, in your backyard, and in lakes or oceans. I love swimming and aqua jogging as part of a comprehensive and personalized health and exercise program.

Weight Training

How many of us have a cute little multi-colored set of hand weights lurking in a cupboard unused, or worse yet, on the floor just waiting to jump out in the middle of the night and stub your toe? It's time to get busy with those weights. Weight training, or strength training, is an absolute requirement for everyone with PCOS. Benefits include:

- Decreased fat mass. Need I say more?
- Improved ability to manage activities of daily living, like picking up a child, carrying groceries, navigating stairs, getting out of a chair, etc.
- Improved bone density – because weight lifting is obviously a weight-bearing activity!
- Decreased injury risk. While increasing your strength, you also increase your body awareness, flexibility, and attention to safety while performing bodily movements. This benefit carries through even when you're not actively lifting weights.
- Promotes body confidence. I don't know about you, but anytime I notice that I've been able to increase my lifting capacity noticeably, I feel pretty proud of myself for that accomplishment. The more you do, or feel capable of doing it, the more likely you are to have those shining moments of pride when you think "my body did THAT!" – and that's a good thing.
- Increased cognitive capacity. Studies have shown increased neuroplasticity in people who weight train. This may also help to reduce depression and anxiety and stave off mental deterioration as you age.
- Increased self-esteem results from developing or improving your skills, seeing changes in your ability to handle the weights, and from the support and feedback of trainers, peers, and friends who see the results of your hard work.
- Improved cardiovascular health, although this is not the focus of weight training.

If you are feeling a little intimidated about the whole idea of weight lifting, you are not alone. It's very important to learn how to lift safely, so that you don't get injured while you're trying to develop strength. Again, the very best way is to get some individualized instruction from a highly qualified personal trainer who can assess your current capabilities and needs, develop a plan, demonstrate correct form, and assist you as you begin to practice.

By "highly qualified," I don't mean "has the best body." I mean, has a long track record of safely training many people, is certified and has appropriate liability insurance, knows first aid and CPR, and listens to your concerns. That person can continue to provide advice and adjust your program as you progress. Make sure you get a good referral from a friend, nutritionist, doctor, or family member. There are probably as many poorly trained (but oh-so-nicely shaped!) trainers out there as there are really good, solid, well-trained, cautious ones. If you can find one who knows anything about PCOS, it's a huge bonus. Otherwise, you will have to give that person some education about what might be different in your body, but don't let the lack of a PCOS savvy trainer hold you back. In this case, it couldn't be truer that "done is better than perfect."

Running

I'm going to briefly go through the benefits of running, although it's not something I like. It tends to be rougher on the body than the above listed activities and may not be appropriate for someone who is carrying a lot of excess weight. Running is favored by many people with mood disorders, often with a complementary yoga program. There seems to be something magical about the combination of the "runner's high" and what happens in yoga practice. Benefits include:

- Building strong bones due to its weight-bearing nature.
- Strengthening muscles.
- Improving cardiovascular fitness.
- Burning a lot of calories.
- Boosting serotonin in your brain to create improved mood.
- Improving self-esteem through the achievement of goals.
- Increasing the brain's release of beta-endorphins, which helps reduce depression.

Other Exercises

Of course, there are many more forms of exercise. I really believe that the best exercises are the ones you will be happy doing for years. You can always change it up along the way, but if you choose an activity you dislike (for me, that would be running), you will not do it consistently, and you won't derive anywhere the near the potential benefit from it. This is all about a long-term strategy that is sustainable, and even enjoyable. Experiment until you figure out what that looks like for you. I did not consider myself athletic at all when I was younger, despite my exercise bulimia, but now I'd say I'm actually moderately athletic, and I really love most of my workouts, and miss them if I can't do them. However, I understand that motivation is difficult, so I'm including some tips on how to increase and maintain your motivation.

Getting Motivated

Getting motivated to start exercising can be a challenge. Here are some ways to get moving NOW (seriously, don't wait until Monday, or the 1st of the month, or after your birthday – just do it now)!

Get medical clearance. It's likely that you're perfectly fine to start exercising, but what if you're not? It's important to make sure that your blood pressure is in a reasonable zone, you don't have any pre-existing injuries that could be exacerbated, and that you don't have blood sugar regulation issues that may require special attention.

Start low and slow. As I described in the walking section, you can literally start with as little as five minutes a day. That means that lack of time is no longer an excuse. As you start to feel some pride in simply getting out there and doing something, your motivation will build, and you will continue work a little harder. Don't worry about meeting any goals except doing it. No need to count steps, chart it out, or record it electronically, unless you find that fun or easy. As you get more confidence, you can start adding more challenging things to your routine.

Get an accountability buddy. Especially in the beginning, it's really helpful to obligate yourself to someone else. You don't want to disappoint your friend who is waiting outside your door at 6:00 a.m. in her tennis shoes, water bottle in hand. You might choose your significant other, a family member, or a work colleague. It really doesn't matter, as long as you commit to keeping one another on track.

Increase time, intensity, and complexity gradually. You don't just jump off a high dive and execute Olympic quality moves on your first try. You don't run a marathon the first time you step it up from a jog to a run. And you don't stand en *pointe* your first day of ballet. We all must begin at the beginning, which is kind of nice if you think about it. Basically, anything you do is better than nothing, and virtually everything you do will be an improvement over the day before. Be mindful of the urge or compulsion to go harder, faster, and longer right away. That's what leads to injuries, exhaustion, burnout, and turning away from a sport that might be absolutely wonderful for you. If you're unsure about what you're planning to do, consult with someone who has more expertise. Get a little supervision or training to make sure your technique is good. Find a club or class where someone else helps keep you safe. That way, you can keep on enjoying the benefits of exercise while limiting your risk of injury.

Pick things you enjoy. As I've said before, if you don't at least sort of like it, you aren't going to do it. In fact, you'll make every excuse in the world NOT to do it. If you hate running, ignore the naysayers who tell you that running is a hundred times more efficient than walking, so why are you wasting your time? Or the ones who tell you that 20 minutes of yoga is "nothing," and you shouldn't even bother if that's all you're going to do. I call B.S. on that right now! Every little bit adds up, and a 20-minute power walk or yoga session can have astonishing benefits, if it's done with consistency. And it's always better than nothing. There are so many different things you can try, there has to be something that you actually think is fun. Maybe it doesn't look like traditional exercise, but it counts anyway: playing catch with your dog, mall walking, heavy-duty yard work, even chasing a bunch of toddlers around – it's all movement, and it's all good.

Set goals. As described above, the goals should be specific to you, measurable (not "walk more," but "walk 20 minutes three times a week" or "Zumba routine at home for 30 minutes, three times a week" instead of "try that Zumba thing"), reasonable, and have some rewards associated with them.

Acknowledge your successes. It's shocking but true that you actually can complete a workout and not post it to social media, but why do people do that anyway? Sure, some of them are bragging, but you can do it for purposes of accountability, adding some external rewards (all those likes and ooohs and aaahs), and to document your own success. After all, if you don't do it, who else will? You're working hard at this, and you deserve some credit for it.

Build in rewards. We're all wired to like treats, pleasure, and rewards, and will engage in behaviors that lead to these good things. Let exercise be one of your paths to reward. Don't make the reward food, but focus on the sense of well-being, increased flexibility and blood flow, sense of accomplishment, or enhanced social life that you develop by walking with a friend as motivators. You might also choose to formalize this, and chart your exercise accomplishments, along with rewards that are meaningful to you. Space the rewards out by a week. For example, if you walk five days out of seven, you get a professional pedicure. If you go to three workout classes at the gym in a week, you get a cool new water bottle. Knowing that there's a prize at the end – even one you give to yourself – is highly motivating.

Be patient but pushy. Know that, if you've never exercised or it's been years, it's going to take you a while to work your way up to doing a lot of anything. Some skills require a bit of practice, like yoga moves, team sports, Pilates, or weight lifting. Do push yourself though; it helps a little, but not enough, to set an initial goal and then just keep meeting that goal over and over. I knew a woman at the gym who would do 60 minutes on the treadmill every day. Every. Single. Day. At first, she lost weight and that was great. And then nothing happened, and it was just boring, and she got an ankle injury. She stopped and never went back. That's not what we're looking for. Achieve, push a little, achieve again, and push some more.

Combatting Boredom

Once you've got a solid start on an exercise routine, you may find yourself getting a little bored, even if you still like an activity. There are many ways to liven things up, switch it around, and get renewed focus and inspiration. Here are a few tips for continued improvement, inspiration, and skill building.

- **Enter a competition!** You don't have to go for a full-scale marathon. There are many events like mini-triathlons (biking, swimming, running/walking) or 5Ks (about three miles). They typically have a built-in support system for training and you may find a new group of friends here.
- **Enter a fundraising walk.** If the sheer joy of competition doesn't do it for you, sign up to walk in the AIDS walk, the walk to end suicide, or the breast cancer walk. Sometimes doing something for others is also a great way to do something for you.
- **Get a private trainer.** It sounds kind of luxurious, and it might be, depending upon whom you choose. But it can also be affordable, and even something that saves you money by reducing your training time, saving you from injury, or introducing you to a creative way of doing something that doesn't require new equipment. You don't have to sign up for months of private training; a few sessions will usually get you over a hump.
- **Become a teacher/coach yourself.** Many people who try popular activities like Tae Bo (okay, flash from the past), yoga, Zumba, etc. get so excited by them that they want to learn more and become teachers themselves. You might also enjoy coaching an activity like softball or soccer, which will force you to study up on technique as you learn how to convey that information to new learners. That can only make you better at what you're doing for yourself.
- **Buy some really cute new workout clothes and shoes.** If you're slumping off to the gym in a ratty old t-shirt that should be banned to the rag pile, and sweats that are now two sizes too

big, you can't see what's happening with your body as you work out, and you're sure not going to like what you see in the mirror. And shoes need to be replaced periodically for both comfort and safety. Cute workout clothes come in all sizes, colors, and configurations. Shopping online may be helpful if you're looking for petites, talls, or plus sizes. And if you need a bathing suit in the dead of winter, online is definitely the way to go.

- **Boast about your accomplishments.** Not in an obnoxious way, but post before and after pictures of yourself somewhere. If you've been keeping quiet about your new workout lifestyle, now's the time to get some positive attention and feedback that will help keep you going.

- **Explore cross training.** When it comes to exercise, I like variety. If you do the exact same thing, for the same amount of time, in the same place, every day, you are going to be bored sooner rather than later. And the exercise will become less effective over time. For optimal health and fitness, you need to cross-train anyway. That sounds fancy, but it's really just making sure you get different activities going that address your needs for strength, flexibility, and cardiovascular health.

- **Try a sport or activity you've never tried before.** Aerial yoga, archery, fencing, adult ballet, salsa dancing, swim team, etc. are all calling you. There's nothing like learning a new skill set to make you appreciate the skills you've already got, and rededicating yourself to comprehensive fitness.

- **Add a team sport.** Whether you loved a sport as a kid or feel like you missed out on that whole team sport thing, now is the time to try it. It could be softball, basketball, or roller derby. Team sports move your body in different ways, add a social element, and require a different type of concentration. There are pick-up games at public parks, adult leagues offered by parks and recreation districts, and company teams.

- **Add a "lifetime"/lifestyle sport, like golf or tennis.** These are the sorts of socially engaged, popular, and well-liked sports that people continue to do well into their 80s and beyond. Social dancing is another one. You can find classes at your local parks and recreation district, community colleges, private clubs or studios, and public courses/courts.

Exercise has powerful physical and psychological benefits, which are of particular importance for women with PCOS. Managing stress, reducing anxiety and depression, and increasing social contact are key benefits of exercise. Exercise is a critical part of any self-care and self-healing process. I hope after reading this that you feel positive and even a little excited about the possibilities that exercise offers.

CHAPTER 19
Putting It All Together

Managing PCOS and its psychological and emotional issues is a lifelong process. You may have different priorities at different times in your life: managing weight, improving depression, dealing with sleep, or getting pregnant. The best approach to all these issues is a holistic and integrative one that includes a well-thought-out approach to selecting quality health care practitioners, supplements, and dietary approaches. It is a process of trial and error, with a lot of steps and experiments. You do need a team of professionals who can help you figure things out and make adjustments as needed.

Now that you know more about what PCOS is, how hormones work, and how important it is to learn to manage it, you also know the critical importance of learning to manage your stress and sleep, as well as diet and exercise. Learning to do your own research, consulting with professionals, and experimenting patiently are the keys to long-term success.

There is nothing easy about PCOS; we have a lot more issues with sleep disorders, eating disorders, mood disorders, and other psychological problems. That doesn't mean it's hopeless, however. There are many tools described in this book, ways to get started, and ways to stay motivated.

Additionally, when do-it-yourself methods aren't working, you've now got a handy reference guide to prescription medications and supplements that help with PCOS-related mood disorders, sleep, and other issues. By starting with "food as medicine," you may be eliminating the need to use supplements or prescription medications, which is even better.

You've also learned several tools that will be helpful for your entire life:

- Practicing acceptance.
- Managing anger.
- Getting proactive.
- Dealing with pain.
- Developing a meditation practice.
- Improving sleep.
- Exercising for health.

Next Steps

Now that you've decided you want to make some serious changes to improve your emotional health (and your physical health in the process), what should you do first?

1. **Start with sleep.** This is the easiest thing to add more of and has the biggest payoff in terms of mood.
2. **Try meditation.** Even a brief daily practice will provide big results.
3. **Go to the doctor.** Get cleared for exercise, get your baseline labs done, or update your lab work, and consult about prescription medications.
4. **Add a little exercise.** Five minutes a day, walking. I promise; it will also have amazing payoffs as far as mood.
5. **Get connected.** As part of PCOS Wellness, I have created a private Facebook group called PCOS Psychology, and I invite you to join the women there. Everyone is supportive and candid about their PCOS experiences.
6. **Make some dietary changes.** You know what you need to focus on here, whether it's cutting refined carbs or simple sugars, increasing protein, or eating consistently. Choose one target at a time and go from there.

7. **Keep researching, seeking, and experimenting.** Our knowledge of PCOS is growing every day; so is research on mental health issues. The more you know, the stronger and healthier you become.

8. **Please review this book on Amazon.** I'm so grateful that you are choosing to take a proactive approach to managing your PCOS. I really appreciate all of your feedback, and love hearing what you have to say. I need your input to make the next version of this book as well as future books better. Please leave me a helpful review on Amazon, letting me know what you thought of the book.

Thank you again for taking the time to read this book. I wish you the best of luck on your PCOS journey.

Appendix: Supplements for PCOS Brain Health

Reminder: Always consult with a well-qualified medical doctor, naturopath, acupuncturist, or dietician before starting or changing any supplements. Like prescription medications, some supplements can have negative side effects, or are not recommended for certain conditions. They should be regularly monitored by your healthcare provider. Always advise all your healthcare providers of the supplements you take, particularly before surgery.

Alpha lipoic acid (ALA) has been demonstrated to be effective in improving insulin sensitivity in women with PCOS and is particularly effective when taken in conjunction with myo-inositol, which is further described below. It also appears to improve nerve conduction, and nerve blood flow. Alpha lipoic acid is a powerful natural antioxidant, and also improves glycemic control in type 2 diabetes (another highly inflammatory condition) patients. The assumption is that improving insulin sensitivity can help decrease inflammation, which affects the brain, so this could be a twofer. Alpha lipoic acid is an antioxidant (more good news for your brain) that actually helps regenerate other antioxidants. It is one of the few supplements that crosses the blood brain barrier, which makes it particularly appealing. If you are taking antipsychotic medications, it can also protect against the common weight gain these medications cause. Typical dosing of alpha lipoic acid is 600 mg to 1,200 mg daily.

Ashwagandha (Indian ginseng) is a plant in the nightshade family (which includes potatoes, tomatoes, and eggplant). It is considered to be one of the most powerful adaptogenic herbs in Ayurvedic medicine. Ashwagandha is reputed to relieve stress, improve immunity, improve fertility, decrease fatigue, increase energy, improve concentration, and protect the brain from the toxic effects of a stressful modern lifestyle. It has also been found to reduce anxiety and depression, stabilize blood sugar, lower cholesterol, act as an anti-inflammatory, and enhance sexual functioning. Can you see why it sounds like it has great potential for helping with PCOS? Ashwagandha is typically taken in capsule form, 600 mg to 1,000 mg twice a day. It can also be consumed as a powder, taken in hot milk, before bedtime.

B-Complex vitamins increase glucose tolerance, prevent nerve damage, and increase glucose metabolism. Vitamin B2 helps to turn the food you eat into energy. Vitamin B3 is a component of the glucose tolerance factor, which is released when you eat. B vitamins also help the liver convert and excrete hormones from the body. Deficiencies in these vitamins can also affect thyroid functioning. There is an ever-growing body of evidence that B vitamins play a key role in mental health. B-Complex vitamins may be useful in preventing or treating diabetic neuropathy, a painful condition in which high blood sugars damage the nerves, resulting in loss of the sensations of touch and temperature.

If you are deficient in the B-Complex vitamins, you could also experience weakness or a lack of muscle coordination, impaired digestion, problems with urinary functioning, and increased vulnerability to infection. Vitamin B5 contributes to fat metabolism and weight loss. Vitamin B6 assists in the manufacture of neurotransmitters (deficiencies contribute to or may cause depression) and it is required for proper synthesis of serotonin, which is implicated in depression. Vitamin B9 (folate) helps with depression and anemia.

Vitamin B12 deficiency occurs in patients who are taking metformin, the most commonly prescribed PCOS medication. It is necessary for optimal nerve functioning and it is also thought that people who are under intense stress (including the chronic stress of post-traumatic stress disorder) suffer from a deficiency of B-Complex vitamins, and "burn through" their B vitamins more rapidly, thus benefitting from supplementation. B vitamins are water soluble, meaning they're excreted in your urine if you take too much (in this case, your urine will likely be shockingly bright yellow). I don't take a B-Complex routinely, but if I'm in a stressful period, I may take a B-complex supplement. I'm not wedded to a particular brand or dosage, because there are so many variations in formulas.

Berberine, an alkaloid found in many herbs, has been described as activating a "metabolic master switch." It helps regulate metabolism and reduce glucose production in the liver, which is one of the problems in PCOS-related insulin resistance. Women with PCOS also have high levels of non-alcoholic fatty liver disease (NAFLD), a potentially very dangerous condition. Berberine helps reduce the bad levels of liver enzymes that are part of NAFLD as well. It has strong anti-bacterial, anti-inflammatory, and immune enhancing properties. It is used as a diabetes treatment in traditional Chinese medicine and may be especially useful for those with poor tolerance to metformin. Side effects may include upset stomach, cramps, and diarrhea, but they are less likely than metformin's side effects, and less severe. I often take Berberine twice a day as a way of boosting the effectiveness of metformin, since I can't tolerate a full dose of metformin. The standard dose of Berberine is 900 mg to 2,000 mg a day, divided into three or four doses; 500 mg taken three times a day may even produce a little weight loss. It should be taken with or shortly after a meal.

Biotin (also known as Vitamin H or Vitamin B7) is a coenzyme that is part of the B-Complex vitamins. Deficiencies may lead to scaly red rashes, cracks in the corners of the mouth, sore tongue, dry eyes, loss of appetite, depression, fatigue, insomnia and more. Biotin contributes to healthy psychological functioning. It helps improve glucose metabolism by stimulating insulin response, synthesizing fats, metabolizing proteins, and improving how the liver processes glucose (improves insulin resistance). A combination of Biotin and Chromium may help support blood sugar improvements and decrease insulin resistance and nerve symptoms related to type 2 diabetes. It's also commonly recommended by both dermatologists and cosmeticians for improving hair growth on the head, as well as weak nails. Reports of side effects are rare.

Biotin is water soluble and best obtained from your diet. Good dietary sources include egg yolks, almonds, cauliflower, cheese, mushrooms, spinach, peanuts, soy nuts, salmon, wheat germ, whole-grain cereals, whole wheat bread, Swiss chard, chicken, and sweet potato. If you need to supplement, dosing varies widely. Adults may take as little as 30 mcg per day of Biotin, although as much as 2 g/day (plus 600 mg of Chromium) may be prescribed for diabetes. As always, start with a low dose and see how you respond, if you choose to supplement.

Calcium is a mineral present mostly in bones and teeth. It also helps the brain use the amino acid tryptophan to manufacture the sleep-inducing substance melatonin, helps release hormones and enzymes, regulates muscle contraction, and plays a role in blood clotting. The melatonin connection explains why a glass of warm milk is a time-honored treatment for insomnia. Dairy products are rich in calcium, but many women with PCOS prefer to avoid dairy. Fortunately, there are other rich non-dairy sources of calcium: spinach, kale, beans, figs, tofu, nuts and seeds, seaweed, collard greens, okra, some fish, and enriched products like orange juice are also good dietary sources of calcium. If you have eliminated dairy from your diet because of allergies, irritable bowel syndrome, or its inflammatory nature, you can also supplement with calcium pills. Calcium is often found bundled with magnesium and zinc, or "cal/mag/zinc." I suggest taking them at bedtime, since they may make you sleepy. A recommended daily dose is around 1,000 mg/day.

Carnitine (L-Carnitine, Acetyl-L-Carnitine) is derived from an amino acid, naturally produced in the body. It can be helpful with muscle disorders, male infertility (and remember, just because you have PCOS doesn't mean that infertility is 100% due to your condition – statistics say it's just as likely to be coming from the other side), chronic fatigue syndrome, diabetes, ADHD, and overactive thyroid, among other conditions. It's important for functioning of the heart, brain, and muscles, and helps the body produce energy. It's widely used in the weight-lifting/bodybuilding world, to improve athletic performance and endurance. It is promoted as a weight loss aid, but scientific evidence is scant. Some people are genetically low in Carnitine, or their Carnitine levels are lowered through use of certain medications or medical procedures (such as dialysis for serious kidney disease). If you are prescribed Depakote (valproic acid), which is used for treatment of bipolar disorder and epilepsy, it may be necessary to counter-balance with Carnitine.

Red meat is one of the primary food sources of Carnitine, although it is also present in fish, poultry, and dairy products, as well as asparagus and wheat bread. Dosing of L-Carnitine varies widely, depending upon the reason you're using it – anywhere from 50 mg/day to 6 g/day may be recommended. So, although your personal trainer may recommend taking L-Carnitine, it's best to get dosing advice from a medical professional. Side effects of L-Carnitine, when taken via injection or by mouth, can include vomiting, upset stomach, heartburn, nausea, diarrhea, and seizures. I have taken L-Carnitine intermittently, because it was recommended as a metabolism booster and weight loss aid, but I don't recommend supplementing unless you've got a solid medical reason to do so.

Cinnamon (cinnamon cassia, cinnamon extract) is a well-known and tasty spice, extracted from the bark of the cinnamon tree, which contains high levels of antioxidants and anti-inflammatories. It has many health benefits, including protecting dental health, freshening breath, fighting viruses and infections, helping with diabetes (lowering blood sugars), protecting the heart, supporting strong brain function, and possibly lowering cancer risk. It is frequently found in oatmeal cookies, gingerbread, sprinkled on your latte, and in mocha-flavored things. Cinnamon extract improves insulin sensitivity in people with diabetes, so presumably it may help improve insulin sensitivity in women with PCOS. It can be consumed as a tea, mixed into smoothies, sprinkled on food, or used in many recipes, but it's difficult to get a consistent and meaningful dose by eating it as a spice, so I think supplements are the best way to go.

The recommended dosage of cinnamon is ½ to one teaspoon per day of powdered cinnamon, the type you get at the grocery store. Feel free to use cinnamon liberally in your food if you enjoy the taste. However, very high doses of cinnamon may be toxic to the liver, and it may lower blood sugar to the degree that, if you are taking hypoglycemic agents (diabetes pills), you may need to lower your dosage. It may also irritate your lips, skin, or mouth. Very rarely is it allergic. I've found that it can be a stomach irritant if you're generally sensitive, but I have taken cinnamon gel capsules twice a day without a problem. I have noticed a distinct improvement in fasting blood sugars, which I check daily, while taking cinnamon as a supplement.

CoQ10 (Coenzyme Q10, Ubiquinone) is found in every cell in your body. CoQ10 is an antioxidant that is used to help the body rebuild cells. Your body makes it, and your cells use it to produce energy. It is necessary for overall cardiovascular health and is depleted when you take statin medications, which are prescribed to reduce cholesterol. If you are taking a statin, you may need to add a CoQ10 supplement, probably around 30 mg to 200 mg per day. It may reduce the muscular pain that is common with some statins and it may speed recovery from exercise. It is also an antioxidant, and it helps the body digest food. CoQ10 is protective of the heart and skeletal muscles as well. Do note that dosing at 100 mg/day can cause insomnia, and 300 mg/day can cause liver toxicity. Good dietary sources of CoQ10 are organ meats (liver, kidneys, and heart), beef, soy oil, sardines, peanuts, and mackerel. I do not take a statin, so I haven't found supplementation with CoQ10 to be necessary. But if you are taking a statin, I think taking it is almost mandatory.

Chromium (forms include **chromium picolinate, chloride, aspartate, amino acid chelates, nicotinate, polynicotinate, and GTF**) is a trace mineral that improves the actions of insulin by serving as a transport aid in your blood stream. The different types are bound to different agents. Chromium polynicotinate, for example, is bound to niacin. Food sources of chromium include liver, mushrooms, wheat germ, chicken breasts, oysters, beets, some wheat products, green beans, potato, prunes, nuts, and some cheeses. Chromium appears to improve insulin regulation in type 2 diabetics and women with PCOS may consider taking 1,000 mcg per day of Chromium to improve insulin sensitivity as well. Because there are so many types, do a little research on which type might serve you best.

Deplin is a prescription supplement (technically a medical food) that helps the body's ability to produce neurotransmitters by addressing nutritional imbalance. It contains L-Methylfolate, an active form of folate. It is typically prescribed in addition to a prescription antidepressant, but it is sometimes used as a standalone treatment for depression, or in combination with other supplements.

Part of the functioning of a healthy brain and body revolves around the process of methylation, which can be impaired in up half the population – and up to 70% of people with depression. This means that you can't activate the folate you need for good mental functioning. This defect or variation in MTHFR (methyltetrahydrofolate reductase) can be detected via a blood test but it is not routinely administered by physicians, so you may have to ask for it. If this gene mutates, you may need a higher level of certain nutrients to achieve optimal health.

If you have the MTHFR gene variation, the best treatment is the supplement called Deplin. It is prescription only, and unfortunately not covered by insurance. Deplin contains L-Methylfolate, a B vitamin, as its active ingredient. It is very difficult to consume the quantity of L-Methylfolate that is necessary for effective treatment via over-the-counter supplements. However, for many people with lifelong depression that have responded only partially to medication, MTHFR and Deplin seem to be the missing piece. I have experienced remarkable improvements taking it myself, and I've observed similar improvements in other patients. If you have long-standing or difficult to treat depression, please explore the MTHFR connection and consider supplementing with Deplin.

DHEA (Dehydroepiandrosterone) is produced by your adrenal system and is a necessary precursor to both estrogen and testosterone. There's some indication that DHEA supplementation can relieve mild to moderate depression. DHEA supplements are made from wild yam or soy. DHEA also counters the action of Cortisol in many tissues. Cortisol is commonly known as the stress hormone – the one that kicks in when your body is freaking out about imminent death. This goes back to the days of being chased by a wooly mammoth. Stress (as well as Cortisol) rises, but then it *should* go right back down when things are working well in the body. But modern life has left a lot of us in a chronically over-stimulated state of stress and distress.

It is theorized that Cortisol is not "processed" adequately in women with PCOS, which increases the body's overall stress load. I agree with this perspective and also believe this is why many women with PCOS report experiencing poor self-control when they are agitated or triggered by something. They may be jumpy, irritable, or quick to become snappish. While low stress tolerance may be the partial result of a bio-chemical issue, it is also something that can be controlled significantly by learning behavior modification techniques, practicing meditation, engaging in measured breathing, and other self-regulation exercises.

In the meantime, supplementation may be helpful. There is one big caveat here: be aware that too much DHEA, taken for too long, can elevate testosterone levels. For many but not all women with PCOS, elevated testosterone is a problem. In fact, for some, testosterone may actually be too low! Testosterone levels can vary over the course of your lifetime, being too high at some points, and too low for optimal functioning at others. I would definitely not go the DIY route on DHEA because side effects include some that are already problematic for women with PCOS, such as oily skin, acne, hair loss, high blood pressure, facial hair, changes in menstrual cycle, deepening of the voice, fatigue, and increased cholesterol levels. Get your hormones tested before supplementing and work with an expert to monitor changes.

DL-Phenylalanine/Phenylalanine is an essential amino acid. The body needs it to make proteins, but cannot produce it, so it must be obtained through food sources or supplementation. Phenylalanine is a precursor for the production of dopamine, which supports mood and endorphins, boosts energy and focus, and combats stress. It may be used for depression, ADHD, chronic pain, osteoarthritis, rheumatoid arthritis, and other conditions. The primary dietary sources of phenylalanine are meat, fish, eggs, cheese, oats, wheat germ, and milk.

It is available in different forms as a supplement: L-Phenylalanine, D-Phenylalanine and DL-Phenylalanine (a combination). Typical doses range from 100 mg to 5,000 mg per day. *Supplements containing Phenylalanine should not be used by people who have been diagnosed with, or are suspected to have, schizophrenia.* Caution should also be used when taking antipsychotic medications for other conditions, such as depression.

Inositol (there are nine different types, but D-Chiro-Inositol and Myo-Inositol are of greatest interest for PCOS patients) is a B-vitamin-like substance found in plants and animals, and also artificially created. It is touted as a near cure-all for women with PCOS. Inositol is important for glucose metabolization, high cholesterol, promoting hair growth, improving ovulation, and decreasing insulin resistance/improving insulin sensitivity. Inositol may also help to relieve the depression that is common in PCOS, as well as panic disorder and obsessive-compulsive disorder. By activating serotonin receptors, it may help improve depression and anxiety, and decrease appetite. Another reputed benefit is that it helps your liver to metabolize fat; this is important because so many women with PCOS have non-alcoholic fatty liver disease.

D-Chiro-Inositol, which improves insulin action, has been shown to affect ovarian function and metabolic factors in women with PCOS, including improving androgen levels, increasing insulin action, lowering triglycerides, reducing blood pressure, improving egg quality, regulating menstrual functioning, and improving ovarian functioning. The body converts Myo-Inositol into D-Chiro-Inositol, but like many things, PCOS bodies don't necessarily do this effectively.

Inositol is available as a stand-alone supplement and there are numerous PCOS-specific formulations. Popular supplements include a powder called Ovasitol, which consists of Myo-Inositol and D-Chiro-Inositol in an optimized 40:1 ratio; Chiral Balance (D-Chiro-Inositol), and Ovaboost (Myo-Inositol). You need both. Myo-Inositol and D-Chiro-Inositol may be taken at 1,200 mg to 2,000 mg/day. Too much D-Chiro-Inositol can actually have the opposite of desired effects. Side effects may include nausea, tiredness, headache, or dizziness. If you don't want to take a supplement, good food sources include fruits, nuts, vegetables, buckwheat, and beans.

Dong Quai (angelica sinesis, "female ginseng") is an herb that is used in traditional Chinese medicine. It is used for menstrual cramps, pelvic pain, low energy, PMS, and menopausal symptoms. It affects estrogen in animals, but it is uncertain if it also affects estrogen in humans. Nonetheless, it is recommended as a good "female" supplement for anyone with menstrual irregularities (thus the name "female ginseng"). It is considered to be a blood purifier, and is helpful for high blood pressure, infertility, psoriasis, ulcers, joint pain, constipation, anemia, and even allergies. It can be taken topically, in a tea, or in a pill/supplement form, as an injection (most commonly in China and Japan) to reduce inflammation, relieve pain, and relax muscles. It may slow blood clotting and increase the risk of bruising and bleeding, so be mindful if you are also taking aspirin, or have a blood clotting disorder. A typical dose is 2,000 mg to 4,000 mg/day, but many practitioners will prescribe much higher doses, particularly for endometriosis, another common complaint of women with PCOS. Dong Quai is one of the first herbal supplements I took when I was attempting to self-medicate my PCOS decades ago; I'm uncertain if it was effective, but I do recommend trying it if it appears suitable.

Essential oils (aromatherapy) have gained tremendous popularity for their purported ability to relieve virtually all manner of ailments, including anxiety, stress, insomnia and depression. Essential oils are the extracts of plant leaves, stalks, rinds, roots, barks, and flowers. They can be used individually or as mixtures for relief of various symptoms. One of the most commonly used for anxiety is lavender, described more fully elsewhere in this chapter. The oils are mixed with a carrier fluid such as oil, alcohol, or lotion, and then inhaled or used topically. The oils stimulate nerves and impulses in the brain that control emotion. Some oils are calming and some are stimulating. Essential oils are typically harmless, but may be problematic for those with allergies or asthma. *They should not be ingested (taken orally) unless you are working with a knowledgeable aromatherapist, as consumption may cause adverse side effects.*

Evening Primrose Oil (EPO, common evening primrose) is an oil derived from the seed of the evening primrose plant. It has long been used by Native Americans for natural healing. It has anti-inflammatory properties that make it effective for eczema, psoriasis, hair and scalp conditions, and acne. It is a good source of Omega-6 essential fatty acids, particularly GLA (Gamma Linoleic Acid).

Another way to get GLA is from borage oil. Taken internally, the body converts the GLA to prostaglandins, which are hormone like compounds that help regulate inflammation associated with pain. It is also useful for arthritis, osteoporosis, ADHD, high cholesterol, heart disease, chronic fatigue, asthma, diabetes, infertility, Reynaud's disease, nerve damage related to diabetes, obesity, premenstrual syndrome, breast pain, endometriosis, and menopause symptoms.

Potential side effects include nausea, diarrhea, headache, and upset stomach. I consider it to be one of the most basic "female supplements" and found profound relief from PMS symptoms in my 20s by taking it daily and doubling the dose for a week before my period (that is, if I could tell when my period was coming!). Up to 3 g per day (1,000 mg three times per day) is considered safe. Even post-menopause, I continue to take 1,000 mg of evening primrose oil daily.

5-HTP (5-Hydroxytryptophan) is something I first learned about in graduate school. I had a colorful and dynamic professor who really liked to play with the brain and do research on himself - and encouraged us students to do so as well. He recommended several supplements that might produce positive mood, stress reduction, and sleep effects, and one of them was 5-HTP, dosed at 50 mg to 150 mg per day, taken in the evening.

A direct precursor to serotonin, 5-HTP helps with mood, relaxation, and sleep. It provides an enhanced feeling of well-being. It is also thought to suppress appetite. As a stressed-out grad student, all of that really sounded great! Unfortunately, for a tiny percentage of patients taking 5-HTP, there will be an adverse reaction, in which you become over-activated and may have problems sleeping. I found out that I was in that group, so I didn't continue with 5-HTP, but I still think it's a great supplement for most people who try it. There are no food sources of 5-HTP, but food sources of tryptophan are useful, because 5-HTP is made from tryptophan, an essential amino acid found in turkey and chicken, milk, potatoes, collard greens, seaweed, sunflower seeds, turnips, and pumpkin.

GABA (Gamma-Aminobutyric acid) is our primary inhibitory neurotransmitter; which helps regulate communication between brain cells. It inhibits or reduces (weakens or slows down) the activity of the neurons or nerve cells. If you are deficient in GABA, you may experience mood disorders, insomnia, or symptoms of PTSD. You may also be low in GABA if carbohydrate cravings are one of your major PCOS symptoms.

GABA has been recommended for anxiety, insomnia, depression, ADD/ADHD, panic attacks, and general nervousness.

Some good food sources of GABA include almonds, liver, broccoli, brown rice, banana, fermented vegetables, sea vegetables, halibut, raw grass-fed cheese, lentils, and oats. For insomnia, dosing is typically 500 mg to 1,000 mg approximately one hour before bed. I am sensitive to GABA and find a low-dose GABA supplement (100 mg) to be extremely useful for easing myself into sleep. For stress, you may also take 100 mg to 500 mg, several times per day (maximum dose of 800 mg/day) or 750 mg split into three doses. It is best consumed on an empty stomach, with a full glass of water. Sublingual tablets may aid in absorption. Side effects are infrequent, and mild, when dosed appropriately. Because it can be highly sedating for some people, I recommend trying it at bedtime before you try taking it in the daytime for anxiety, or you might find yourself napping during the day!

Ginger is a root in the same family as turmeric. Like turmeric, it contains curcumin, which is anti-inflammatory, antioxidant, antiviral, antibacterial, and antifungal. Ginger increases motivation, memory, and attention. Ginger may also improve neurotransmitter balance, health, and function, reduce brain aging and inflammation, and improve diabetes. It is widely used as a culinary spice and for its medicinal qualities, particularly in India and Asia. It is available as a whole, fresh root which must be peeled and shredded or chopped, ginger juice, powdered ginger, sliced, candied ginger, and as pre-chopped jarred/canned ginger.

The most well-known medicinal use of ginger is as a digestive aid/nausea reducer. It's also been used to treat arthritis, muscle aches, pain, cramps, colds, flu, sore throat, asthma, and diabetes. It's an excellent anti-inflammatory and may ward off the neurological effects of diabetes (remember that nearly half of us will develop diabetes by the age of 40). It contains over 100 compounds – 50% of which are antioxidants! Given the high number of women with PCOS who report "brain fog" as a symptom, as well as anxiety and depression, I think trying ginger is a low-risk way to get some rapid improvement. It's also quite tasty.

The easiest way to start consuming ginger is to find a good quality herbal ginger tea or simply slice or grate some fresh ginger into a cup of boiling water. A little powdered ginger dissolved in hot water serves the same function. It has a bit of a spicy sweet quality to it. It is often found mixed with lemon, in chai, in items such as flavored waters and iced teas, and kombucha. And, of course, there are powdered ginger supplements in capsule form. Gingerbread and ginger cookies, while tasty, come with a high load of sugar and refined flour, so they're not the best sources of ginger. Do not take more than 4 g of ginger per day (1 g to 3 g is typical), as it could cause heartburn or overly thin the blood.

Gymnema Sylvestre is a woody shrub, the leaves of which are used to make medicine. It decreases the absorption of sugar from the intestine, slowing the transport of glucose to the bloodstream, which can help regulate blood sugar levels. It may also increase the amount of insulin in the body, and even increase the growth of pancreatic cells. In Ayurvedic medicine, it is traditionally used for sugar regulation, diabetes, hypoglycemia, cholesterol, as a laxative, and for weight reduction. It is thought to reduce sugar cravings by dulling the taste for sweets. Gymnema should be stopped two weeks before surgery. It is strong enough that, if taken with diabetes drugs such as metformin, it could lower blood sugar too much, so dose mindfully. Dosing is not standardized, but typically varies from 3.5 ml to 11 ml of liquid extract.

Kava (Piper methysticum) is a medicinal root, typically consumed in beverage or supplement form, which is found the Pacific Islands. It has a calming effect, which produces similar brain changes to the prescription drug Valium. It is taken for anxiety, stress, restlessness, and insomnia. *However, kava has caused liver failure in previously healthy people.* Additionally, it should not be consumed with prescription psychotropic medications or alcohol. Given the propensity towards non-alcoholic fatty liver disease in women with PCOS, I heartily recommend staying away from this one.

Lavender (Lavandula angustifolia) is a beautiful, abundantly occurring herb that can be used in many forms, including teas (avoid consuming the oils), capsules, sprays, sachets, and essential oils. The leaves and oils are used medicinally. Many people find lavender relaxing. Lavender reduces anxiety, helps regulate stress responses, promotes restful sleep, and supports positive mood. It is a versatile substance that may also help with pain, gastrointestinal distress, infections, acne, migraine, to promote menstruation, and to decrease restlessness. Taking lavender by mouth, however, can cause constipation, headaches, and increased appetite.

Lavender can be applied to the skin for hair loss, but can cause skin irritation in sensitive individuals. Since many women with PCOS become depressed and anxious about their hair loss, lavender might be a good and relatively harmless starting point for hair loss treatment and the related mood changes. Mild to moderate anxiety can be helped with oral lavender. Lavender combined with sedative drugs for sleep may result in too much of an effect (too much sleepiness). It is also recommended to stop using lavender two weeks before surgery, because it may slow down the central nervous system too much.

L-Glutamine (Glutamine) is an amino acid found in the body naturally. It helps with gut, immune and stress issues. It is used for many things, including digestive conditions, depression, hypoglycemia, moodiness, irritability, anxiety, insomnia and enhancing exercise performance. L-Glutamine helps combat cravings for sweets and starches, and may be especially helpful combined with chromium. Good food sources of glutamine include beef, chicken, fish, dairy, eggs, cabbage, spinach, carrots, wheat, papaya, celery, kale, and fermented foods. As a supplement, dosing is typically at 500 mg to 1,500 mg/day, spread throughout the day in three equal doses. As much as 40 g per day is considered safe.

Lithium Orotate. Lithium, you say? Isn't that the stuff they give bipolar people? Yes and no. Lithium, sometimes combined with Valproic Acid, is indeed a highly effective treatment for bipolar disorder. But Lithium is also a naturally occurring salt that assists in proper functioning of enzymes, hormones, and vitamins. It is a neuro-stabilizer that many people find useful for mood regulation, balancing both anxiety and depression. It may also help regenerate brain cells, improve blood sugar metabolism, insomnia, hormonal issues, and digestive issues.

It is found in hot springs, seawater, ground water, vegetables, grains, other plant sources, and some meats. Keeping in mind that correlation is not necessarily causation (just because it appears simultaneously doesn't mean it's absolutely linked), there is increasing evidence that, as Lithium has been increasingly filtered out of our water supply, there has been an increase in psychiatric disorders. Low levels of Lithium in local water supplies are associated with increased suicide, homicide, and arrests for drug use.

Lithium Orotate is available as an over-the-counter supplement, but it must be taken judiciously. Some professionals recommend against using it as a supplement because of the potential for side effects including nausea, fine tremor, frequent urination, diarrhea, thirst, dizziness, muscle weakness, and fatigue. It leaves the body quickly and a maximum of 20 mg/day, split morning and evening, is recommended. It should be started at 5 mg/day and increased gradually. I added 20 mg/day of lithium orotate to my supplement regiment a few years ago and I feel that it has been very helpful in terms of calming my PCOS-related anxiety and irritability. *It is also recommended that, if you supplement with lithium, you have periodic blood tests, at least in the beginning, to ensure that you do not develop lithium toxicity.* In other words, please use Lithium supplements under the close supervision of a qualified medical professional.

L-Theanine/Theanine is an amino acid that is used to boost focus and concentration as well as promote relaxation without sedation. L-Theanine is a slightly different molecular formulation than just Theanine, and that's what we're looking for. It is considered an adaptogen, in that it both enhances brain function and helps your body deal with stress. It has been found to increase alpha brainwave activity. Alpha brainwaves help you feel relaxed without actually feeling sleepy, so you feel calm, alert, and focused.

Consuming L-Theanine increases the production of GABA and dopamine, neurotransmitters that are associated with calming. It works by reducing sympathetic nervous system activation when you are under stress and can be particularly useful when consumed before a known stressful event, such as a test or speaking engagement. It is found exclusively in black, green, and white teas, and is about 2.5% of the dry weight of the tea leaves. Interestingly, it is synergistic with caffeine, meaning that it actually has a calming effect when consumed with caffeine, and the mental boost is better. Note that "herbal" teas are not actually tea, and therefore contain no Theanine. Green tea contains the most L-Theanine. Because it also contains some caffeine (nowhere near the caffeine in coffee), you don't necessarily want to consume endless quantities.

Theanine can also decrease blood pressure. It can help reduce anxiety and contribute to a more relaxed, yet alert, mental state. It is typically dosed at 100 mg to 200 mg twice daily if used in supplement form, which is probably a lot more than you would get from drinking green or black tea all day, as a cup of tea contains anywhere from 3.8 mg to 5.7 mg of L-Theanine. I recommend starting with tea before trying it as a supplement.

L-Tryptophan is an essential amino acid that must be acquired from food, as the body doesn't make it. After L-Tryptophan is absorbed, it converts to 5-HTP, and then to serotonin. It is useful for depression, mood swings, tension, irritability, insomnia, and premenstrual dysphoric disorder. It is typically dosed at 500 mg to 1,500 mg per day, taken by about 10:00 p.m. Over the years, L-Tryptophan supplements have had a mixed reputation. Potential side effects include gastrointestinal distress, visual blurring, drowsiness, and muscular weakness. Taking L-Tryptophan while taking an antidepressant may cause you to have too much serotonin, which can be dangerous. While it is treated as a supplement, this is powerful stuff and best taken with the guidance of a healthcare professional.

L-Tyrosine is another one of the amino acids, the building blocks of protein. It is made from phenylalanine, discussed below. It has been used for ADHD, narcolepsy (involuntarily falling asleep), depression, stress, premenstrual syndrome, Parkinson's and Alzheimer's diseases, chronic fatigue syndrome, heart disease, low libido and as an appetite suppressant, to list some of its many uses. It improves mental performance and alertness, such as before taking a test, and increases alertness in people who have been sleep-deprived. Good food sources are dairy products, fish, eggs, meat, nuts, beans, wheat, and oats. Supplemental Tyrosine, commonly dosed at 150 mg/day with a maximum daily dose of 500 mg to 2,000 mg, is generally considered safe. Some people may experience side effects such as headache, nausea, fatigue, heartburn or joint pain.

Magnesium is a calming, relaxing mineral that has been shown to decrease insulin resistance and help keep blood sugar levels healthy. It is often deficient in our diets, and stress further depletes magnesium, which usually serves to regulate cortisol. Magnesium and other trace minerals are part of the complex underlying picture of PCOS. People with metabolic syndrome, essentially many PCOS patients, have a much greater likelihood of being low in Magnesium. My thinking is that if you have PCOS, you have Magnesium deficiency.

Magnesium is critical to the functioning of every aspect of your body. It contributes to healthy nerve function, heart regulation, and immune system functioning, among other things. It helps regulate the nervous system, helps you cope with stress, helps your cells make energy, improves insomnia, relaxes muscles, may reduce cortisol, and decreases anxiety, nervousness, restlessness, and irritability. It is also helpful in activating Vitamin D in your body. It enhances insulin secretion, promotes sleep serves as a general systemic relaxant and is anti-inflammatory in nature. Magnesium can act at the blood/brain barrier to prevent stress hormones from entering the brain (therefore it is protective for the brain).

A deficiency may play a role in anxiety and depression, as well as those pesky sugar and carb cravings. Birth control pills also deplete Magnesium while the consumption of refined carbohydrates and excess sugar may increase your need - which is one more reason why dietary management of PCOS is so important. Deficiencies may result in cardiac arrhythmias, depression, headaches, seizures, Ataxia (coordination problems and gait/ walking abnormality), psychosis, irritability, and muscle cramps.

You can get Magnesium from dark leafy greens, nuts, seeds, seafood, beans, whole grains, avocados, yogurt, bananas, dried fruit, and dark chocolate. Yes, dark chocolate is a great source of Magnesium! But a "dose" is about 1 oz. Generally speaking, foods that are high in fiber are also high in Magnesium (nature is pretty cool that way). And more good news – coffee is high in magnesium!

The current recommended daily value for Magnesium is 400 mg, but this is highly personal and you should experiment until you find what works best for your body. If you have irritable bowel syndrome or related gastrointestinal diseases, be especially mindful of the potential for diarrhea. I take a small dose of ionic liquid Magnesium periodically as a sleep aid. This form can also be added to your day's drinking water supply, so that you get a very small steady dose.

Another way to increase your intake is via Epsom salts in your bath so that it is absorbed through the skin. This is a great two-for-one, in that a warm bath is almost always deeply relaxing. There is also something called Magnesium Oil, which isn't actually "oil", that you spray on your skin and rub in. That can be sticky and messy, but it's worth a try if you haven't been able to consume it successfully. There are also topical Magnesium Creams you can rub in to your skin.

Magnesium supplements are available in several forms, including Magnesium Citrate, and Magnesium Oxide. Choose whatever is readily available and see how it works; it is quite inexpensive. You may notice a positive effect from only 200 mg/day. If you are not getting enough dietary Calcium, then taking a combination supplement which has about double the Calcium (two-to-one ratio) could be desirable – but if you're consuming too much Calcium, that can also alter Magnesium levels.

As noted above, excessive Magnesium can also contribute to gastrointestinal distress, including diarrhea. If you are already feeling the effects of metformin, start slowly – very slowly – when adding magnesium to your diet. If you have kidney disease, bowel obstruction, abnormal heart rhythms, or Myasthenia Gravis, consult with your physician before supplementing with Magnesium. It may not be suitable for you. It can also interfere with the absorption of some medications, including antibiotics, so again, double-check with your doctor or pharmacist.

Marijuana (Cannabis, CBD, THC) is a plant that is grown for both its psychoactive as well as medicinal properties. Due to the varying and rapidly changing legal nature of medical Marijuana in different locales, I've included it in both the prescription and non-prescription sections of this book. Marijuana contains cannabinoids called cannabidiol (CBD) and tetrahydrocannabinol (THC). The THC is the part that gets you high, but it's also useful in modulating pain, nausea, seizures, and inflammation. CBD is thought of as the more "medical" part of the plant, but our understanding of how it works, how much is useful, and how much is dangerous is also changing rapidly.

Conventional thinking, which focused almost exclusively on the intoxicating effects of THC, holds that Marijuana induces paranoia, lethargy, and anxiety/agitation, but newer information indicates that THC plus CBD in the right ratios, or CBD exclusively, *may* help with PTSD, depression, anxiety, bipolar disorder, and sleep disorders. If marijuana is legal in your state or country, it's worth exploring the CBD-dominant preparations (vapors, topicals, oils, and other edibles) to see if they may offer some relief for your symptoms. While the legal status of Marijuana has left research deficits, there is a great deal of research in the pipeline right now, and the potential is exciting to contemplate.

Melatonin is a hormone that is produced by the pineal gland. It is affected by light, and regulates sleep and wakefulness. You may be familiar with it as a tool to help reset your body clock while travelling. Very small amounts of it are found in whole foods like grain, fruit, meat, and vegetables, but it is generally taken as a supplement. If everything in your body is working well, Melatonin levels should begin to rise in the mid-to-late evening, remain high most of the night, and then decrease in the morning.

The most commonly recommended dose is 3 mg, taken at bedtime, and you can safely take up to 5 mg/night, although I've seen dosage recommendations ranging from 0.2 mg to 20 mg/day. Here's the surprise though: according to sleep experts, you only need 0.25 mg to 0.5 mg to trigger sleep, and that dose should be taken three to four hours before bedtime. Play with the timing though; I find that taking it about two hours before bed is the right timing for me. But if you have trouble sleeping through the night, it may also be useful to also take a small dose at bedtime, which sends a mid-sleep cycle message to your body to keep sleeping. As a bonus, Melatonin is also a powerful antioxidant. Side effects include vivid dreams and morning grogginess. Because Melatonin is a hormone, it is preferable to take it only as needed.

Milk Thistle (silymarin, Mary thistle, holy thistle) is a flowering herb related to the daisy and ragweed family. It is an antioxidant and anti-inflammatory. It may help with infertility, depression, non-alcoholic fatty liver disease (NAFLD), cholesterol levels and lowering blood sugars. Liver "cleansing" and regeneration are the most common uses of Milk

Thistle and it is considered to be especially helpful to women with insulin resistance. But it can cause gastrointestinal side effects, such as diarrhea or nausea. There is also a concern that milk thistle may act like or with estrogen, which may actually be a good thing for women with PCOS, because it helps break down and release excess estrogen. A typical daily dose is 200 mg. I don't consider it a key supplement for the treatment of depression, but I like the overall package of benefits for those of us with NAFLD and insulin resistance. Be mindful of Milk Thistle if you have an allergy to ragweed.

N-Acetyl Cysteine (NAC) is derived from the amino acid L-Cysteine. It is used to make glutathione, one of the body's antioxidants, and has significant anti-inflammatory effects. Although it is not considered a key supplement for depression, it has some antidepressant effects. Because of its other tremendous benefits, I consider it a necessary component of any comprehensive supplementation program for women with PCOS, who have higher levels of oxidative stress, so antioxidants are especially important. Studies show a positive effect for reducing symptoms of obsessive-compulsive disorder, including skin picking and hair pulling.

The broader benefits for PCOS include: improved insulin sensitivity, lowering testosterone and free androgen levels, improving menstrual regularity, increasing frequency of ovulation, supporting egg quality and raising progesterone levels. It also helps to lower cholesterol levels and is widely recommended for PCOS patients because it may help with NAFLD. The dosage is 1.6 g to 3 g/day (maximum of 7 g/day), and you may need to be on the higher end of this range if you are overweight. It can cause gastrointestinal side effects, rashes, and headaches.

Omega-3 Fatty Acids (EPA/DHA). I think of these as the brain fats, because they're so good for brain health. Technically, they are long-chain fatty acids, comprised of Eicosapentaenoic Acid (EPA) and Docosahexaenoic Acid (DHA). The body cannot make essential fatty acids; we must obtain them from our diet. So, when your mother said: "fish is brain food," she was giving sound medical advice. People who eat more fish and other foods high in Omega-3s have lower levels of depression. Fish oil may help antidepressants work better and improve bipolar symptoms. These fatty acids help your neurotransmitters work well, increase serotonin levels, support immune function and blood clotting, and contribute to cell growth and cellular membrane structure.

We should have an approximately one-to-one ratio of Omega-3 to Omega-6 in our diet, yet the average American consumes up to 17 times more Omega-6 fatty acids than Omega-3 fatty acids, mostly from vegetable oils. In fact, it is estimated that soybean oil (found in innumerable processed products) is the source of up to 11% of the calories Americans consume! Of even greater interest to women with PCOS, the body constructs hormones from the Omega-6 fatty acids – the types of hormones that tend to increase inflammation, blood clotting, and cell proliferation, while Omega-3 fatty acids decrease those functions. We are always looking to decrease inflammation in women with PCOS, as the inflammatory effects on body and brain are profound.

Supplementing with high quality fish oil is helpful for brain health, reducing depression, and lowering cholesterol. Fish oil supplements can go rancid easily and may not be sourced from the healthiest fish. I advise seeking out fish oil from wild/organic fish, possibly refrigerated, and definitely from a source that has rapid product turnover. Salmon oil is a common source, but krill oil or cod liver oil can be other good sources.

Food sources include fish, of course (eating fish two to three times per week has been recommended, but we also must be mindful of cumulative mercury loads), chia seeds, walnuts, fish roe (eggs), soybeans, eggs, enriched dairy foods and spinach. Flaxseeds (ground, not whole) or flax seed oil also contain the Omega-3s and may be a good substitute if you are vegetarian, allergic to or dislike fish. If you choose to supplement, look for at least 500 mg to 1,000 mg (1 g) of EPA plus DHA in your daily dose. Therapeutic doses may be much higher – as high as 3 g to 6 g/day.

Probiotics/psychobiotics are anti-inflammatory microbes that affect the gut in a positive way. Psychobiotics may be a term you haven't heard before; they are mind-altering probiotics used in the same way as other supplements to improve mental functioning. Most of your neurotransmitters are produced in your gut, which makes gut health critical for mental health. As yet, there are no standard prescriptions of probiotics for mental health disorders, but they offer interesting possibilities. Probiotics are an emerging area of interest for regulating brain health and mood disorders, as poor gut health is implicated in depression and anxiety. They can decrease stress signaling in the body and increase the transformation of tryptophan to serotonin in the brain. Psychological improvements have been noted with anxiety, depression and decreases in negative thinking.

There are many probiotics. Some of the most common include lactobacillus plantarum, lactobacillus acidophilus, lactobacillus brevis, bifidobacterium lactis, and bifodobacterium longum. Good food sources include most fermented foods, such as sauerkraut, kim chi, yogurt, kefir, pickles, and kombucha. Supplements are widely available and may be useful to increase the diversity of Probiotics that you consume, but I recommend starting with increasing the dietary sources. It is possible to overdo it with Probiotics, particularly if you have SIBO (small intestine bacterial overgrowth).

Rhodiola Rosea (golden root) is a plant, the root of which is used as a medicine. It is often recommended for depression, diabetes, and liver damage prevention. It reportedly is of great use in fat burning (particularly belly fat), enhancing energy, lowering cortisol, improving depression, and brain boosting power. Elevated cortisol can lead to poor blood glucose stability, abdominal weight gain, thyroid issues, hormonal imbalance, memory issues, and decreased immunity. Other benefits of Rhodiola include improved work performance, increased stamina, reduced anxiety, heightened ability to resist toxins and environmental stress, and decreased insomnia and fatigue. Rhodiola stabilizes adrenal hormones and helps with the production of serotonin. It can help improve your ability to handle stress, improve concentration, and provide an immune and energy boost.

Rhodiola increases the sensitivity of the neurotransmitters serotonin and dopamine, both of which increase memory, focus, pleasure, and mood. It may also help decrease food cravings. Typically, it is taken twice a day at 250 mg to 500 mg per dose. I have taken low-dose Rhodiola on and off for many years, and it is considered likely to be safe when taken for up to 10 weeks at a time.

SAMe (Sam-E, S-Adenosyl-Methionine) is formed naturally in the body, as well as in laboratories. It is involved in the creation, activation, and breakdown of hormones, proteins, lipids, and some medications. People who don't make enough SAMe naturally may benefit from taking it as a supplement. It has been used to treat a variety of psychiatric conditions, along with osteoarthritis and several other inflammatory conditions. A partial list of conditions treated with SAMe include anxiety, heart disease, fibromyalgia, arthritis, tendonitis, bursitis, low back pain, Alzheimer's disease, chronic fatigue syndrome, liver disease, PMS, pre-menstrual dysphoric disorder, Parkinson's disease, ADHD, multiple sclerosis, spinal cord injury, seizures, and migraines. For our purposes, the usefulness of SAMe as an anti-depressant is the most important, but if you have any of these other conditions, you may experience more benefits.

It is available over-the-counter, and broadly used in Europe since at least the 1970s, in lieu of pharmaceutical antidepressants. It can be administered intravenously or injected as a shot, although I haven't found it used that way in the United States. It may be better tolerated than St. John's Wort and is unlikely to cause any side effects in my experience, except perhaps mild nausea. At higher doses, it may occasionally cause gas, vomiting, constipation, sweating, dizziness, or nervousness. It acts quickly, with benefits noticeable in as few as 48 hours, especially compared with antidepressants, which typically take six weeks. And unlike prescription antidepressants, there's no problem starting and stopping it.

It is typically sold in 200 mg increments, and you can safely take up to 1,600 mg/day. It is often enough to take 200 mg/day, although many patients will require 400 mg/day, or more to feel their best. At higher doses, the risk of gastrointestinal distress increases slightly. Interestingly, it can also give a little buzz or lift to people not suffering from depression, kind of like a natural upper. It does tend to be a little expensive, which is a negative.

SAMe can cause dangerous highs (hypomania or mania) in people with bipolar disorder. Dosing is best regulated by a knowledgeable practitioner rather than on your own. SAMe can safely be used with prescription antidepressants, or in combination with St. John's Wort, but the effects are additive (meaning, you could end up with too much serotonin in your brain), so again, work with a healthcare professional to make sure you aren't overdoing it. Basically, just because it's available over-the-counter, treat it as you would any other medication – with caution. Over the years, I have had good experiences using SAMe independently at doses of up to 800 mg/day, and in combination with prescription antidepressants at about 400 mg to 600 mg/day. Many of my clients have tried SAMe with similarly good results.

St. John's Wort, which is derived from a plant, has been used for centuries for health purposes. According to the Mayo Clinic, St. John's Wort may be as effective as tricyclic antidepressants and the more commonly prescribed selective serotonin uptake inhibitors (SSRIs). It is useful for mild to moderate depression, but it can cause serious interactions with other herbs, supplements, and prescription medication.

Like SAMe, St. John's Wort is commonly prescribed in Europe for depression, but it is not a proven therapy for depression. There are numerous studies, yet the results continue to be mixed. For some patients, it is highly effective, has little to no side effects, and may even boost libido (a potential benefit for women with PCOS), plus it improves sleep. Like SSRIs, it appears to inhibit reuptake of serotonin, and possibly also noradrenaline, dopamine, and GABA activity, which makes it a pretty comprehensive solution to depression issues. There are no natural food sources of St. John's Wort.

For depression, it is commonly dosed at 300 mg, taken three times a day, possibly lowering to 300 mg to 600 mg once a day after relief is obtained. Like Sam-E, positive effects may be noticeable within days instead of the weeks required for SSRIs, and it can be easily stopped and started. Pharmaceutical antidepressants typically take about three weeks to kick in, and about six weeks to become fully effective, and you must titrate on and off them to avoid problems. St. John's Wort does carry the potential for some side effects, such as rashes, tremor, confusion, muscle stiffness, allergy, and gastrointestinal distress. Taking St. John's Wort can also weaken the effects of prescription medications, including antidepressants and birth control pills. *Too much St. John's Wort taken with prescription antidepressants can create a dangerous condition known as serotonin syndrome, which is potentially life threatening.* Because SAMe functions much the same way, with a better side effect profile, I would almost always say that SAMe is a better choice for mild to moderate depression.

Triphala is an Ayurvedic concoction comprised of three fruits that support functioning of the liver, immune system and respiratory system. It removes toxins and helps to maintain a healthy weight. It is recommended more than any other Ayurvedic product. It cleanses and detoxifies gently, while also nourishing and replenishing the system. Studies indicate improved gastrointestinal health, and better cholesterol levels. Triphala may help reduce food cravings by providing a balance of the taste sensations including sour, sweet, astringent, pungent and bitter notes. It is traditionally consumed as a tea (1/2 teaspoon of Triphala powder to a cup of hot water), taken on an empty stomach before bed or first thing in the morning. For easier consumption, it is also available as a liquid extract. As a detoxifier/cleansing agent, you may experience looser bowel movements when taking Triphala, so start with a small amount and see how you feel.

Turmeric/Curcumin comes from the underground stems of a plant in the ginger family. It is a beautiful deep golden yellow (which is also how American mustard gets its color) and is commonly used as a spice in Indian cooking. It has a pungent, bitter, aromatic quality with a scent of orange or ginger. The most active medicinal part of Turmeric is Curcumin, which is a powerful antioxidant and anti-inflammatory. In Ayurvedic medicine, it may be used as a treatment for laryngitis, bronchitis and diabetes. When people consume turmeric regularly, as in India, there are lower rates of Alzheimer's disease. It may reduce pain and joint swelling from arthritis, have protective effects against cancer and improve autoimmune conditions.

Taking 400 mg to 600 mg of Turmeric in capsules two to three times a day is a common use. Stand-alone Curcumin is also available, and I believe that the whole food form is always the best option. It's hard for me to get enough through food, so I usually take 500 mg, twice per day. It should ideally be accompanied by some black pepper for absorption. In addition to Indian food, you might try it with eggs, roasted vegetables, rice, greens, soups, smoothies, or teas. A classic health concoction called "Golden Milk" is made from two cups of milk, a teaspoon of Turmeric, some cinnamon, a teaspoon of raw honey or maple syrup, black pepper and a dash of ginger powder, which is heated and blended well, and consumed before bed. Since most of us aren't eating turmeric-heavy Indian food every day, supplementation is a solid option. Turmeric may cause stomach upset, heartburn, or interference with elimination of some medications including chemotherapy drugs.

Valerian root is an herbal medication made from the root of the valerian plant. Despite the name sounding like the prescription Benzodiazepine medication that is very relaxing, Valium, it is not related (other than that both are thought to affect the level of GABA amino acids in the brain). However, it does act as a sedative on the nervous system and brain. It's been found to be helpful for insomnia and other sleep disorders, anxiety, asthma, nervousness and excitability, tension headaches, migraines and upset stomach. It's also used for depression, ADHD, joint pain, cramps, menopause, hot flashes, and chronic fatigue syndrome.

There are no food sources of Valerian. While sleeping pills work "instantly," it may take up to a month of consistent use before Valerian helps with sleep or insomnia issues. The dosing for insomnia is 400 mg to 900 mg of Valerian extract, 30 minutes to two hours before bedtime. Some Valerian-containing products will include lemon balm extract and hops, which can also help with sleep. For PMS, Valerian can be taken three times a day for the length of two menstrual cycles. Valerian can have contradictory effects, meaning it causes insomnia in some people. It may also increase excitability or nervousness.

Vitamin C (Ascorbic Acid) helps the body form and maintain connective tissue, such as bone and skin. It helps repair tissues and may neutralize the effects of nitrites. A powerful antioxidant, it may help mitigate kidney damage. It has been much touted for improving immunity, such as in cancer or the common cold. It helps the body absorb iron and is a powerful antioxidant. Vitamin C also protects against heart disease and can decrease total cholesterol and triglycerides. It may help raise progesterone in women with PCOS, which needs to be considered in the context of your individual body.

It's now clear that it can reduce stress on our bodies and brains as well - people who have high levels of Vitamin C are more resilient to the effects of stress. Vitamin C reduces the secretion of cortisol, which triggers the "fight or flight" response in our bodies and is constantly over-triggered by the stressors of modern life. Frequent bursts of cortisol will eventually wear down the body, reduce memory, impair learning and make people more likely to experience clinical depression.

Vitamin C is found abundantly in fruits and vegetables. There is little to no Vitamin C in animal food. Vitamin C is destroyed by heat and cooking, so the raw factor is important here. Food sources of Vitamin C are abundant and include fresh raw fruits and vegetables such as oranges, chili peppers, red and green bell peppers, Brussels sprouts, kale, broccoli, cauliflower, pineapple, kiwi, strawberries, guava, grapefruit, tomatoes, asparagus, apples, berries, spinach, potatoes, and parsley.

Vitamin C deficiency symptoms include fatigue, muscular aches and weakness, bleeding gums and leg rashes. Recommendations for how much Vitamin C to take vary enormously, from 25 mg to 2,000 mg/day, with higher doses recommended during periods of acute stress when your body "burns" it more rapidly. Nobel Prize winner and researcher Linus Pauling famously took 2,000 mg/day (or more), yet the current recommended daily allowance is 60 mg to 75 mg/day. Vitamin C is a water-soluble vitamin, which means it is easily purged from your system, so it's difficult to take too much. Many people think that powdered Vitamin C/Ascorbic Acid is better absorbed, but either powder or capsule form is fine. Taking more than 2,000 mg/day can contribute to formation of kidney stones. If you have diarrhea or nausea, you'll know you've "overdosed."

Vitamin D3. The two critical balancing agents in sleep regulation are Melatonin (see above) and Vitamin D3. If one or both levels are off, your sleep will also be off. Melatonin tells your body to go to sleep, and Vitamin D3 tells your body to wake up. It also has antidepressant effects. It's typically produced when you are exposed to the sun (about 20 – 30 minutes per day will do it). It then converts to the vitamin in your body. If you're wearing enough sunscreen though, it's unlikely that you're getting the sun exposure you need to be healthy. Physicians now routinely check Vitamin D levels. If you are deficient (anything under 30), your doctor will likely prescribe 50,000 units to be taken once a week until your levels return to normal.

You can easily supplement with over-the-counter Vitamin D3 oil/gel capsules, which typically are 2,000 units each. Many people routinely take anywhere from 2,000 units to 10,000 units/day to maintain a Vitamin D level at around 60. Having a level around 60 – 70 is a "functional medicine" preferred level, and anything higher may be tending toward a dangerous level.

The role of Vitamin D in diabetes and PCOS is still being researched. It is well known though that Vitamin D contributes to bone health, cardiovascular health, and immune functioning, which can be compromised by diabetes. Vitamin D supplementation may improve insulin sensitivity, which is reduced in PCOS. Since Vitamin D3 is a hormone, it stands to reason that it will be a continuing topic of interest and evolving thought; it's important to check in with your medical treatment team periodically about current recommendations.

Vitamin E is an antioxidant that helps with the production and repair of skin. It may be useful also in lowering the risk of Alzheimer's, decreasing anxiety and stress, and improving depression. Vitamin E is an oil/fat-soluble vitamin, which means that you must be more careful consuming it, as it is not as easily purged from your body as the water-soluble vitamins. Therefore, high-dose Vitamin E is not recommended. Food sources are preferable, and include meats, poultry, eggs, wheat germ, plant oils, avocado, broccoli, papaya, apricots, olives, dark leafy greens, hazelnuts, pine nuts, peanuts, almonds, sunflower seeds, basil, parsley, and oregano. If you choose to supplement, seek consultation, and start low and slow.

Vitex (Chasteberry or Chaste Tree) is a traditional herbal medication made from the dried fruit of the Chasteberry Tree. It inhibits production of prolactin. Women with PCOS often have high levels of prolactin. Vitex stimulates ovulation and promotes menstrual regularity. It also contains opioid-like compounds that can reduce PMS, stress, sleep problems, and anxiety. Vitex can be powerful when used correctly, but it's among the supplements I wouldn't use without consulting with a herbal medicine expert, as it can have numerous negative side effects, including acne, headache, rash, stomach upset, weight gain and menstrual bleeding.

Zinc is an essential trace mineral that has been found to be low in individuals with depression, particularly women. It works in conjunction with Copper, and an excess of or imbalance of Copper can leave you depleted of Zinc, which activates GABA receptors in the brain. Therefore, Zinc is calming and sedating. It is an anti-inflammatory and anti-depressant in its own right.

The more depressed you are, the lower your level of Zinc is likely to be. Low Zinc levels also decrease immunity and increase inflammation in the body. Pancreatic beta cells (part of insulin resistance and diabetes) also use Zinc, so this is of particular interest to women with PCOS. It plays a part in regulating the body's response to stress. Zinc works with more than 300 other enzymes in the body, but the highest quantity of Zinc is found in our brains. Low levels of Zinc can lead to ADHD, seizures, aggression, problems with learning and memory, and even violence. And when we are highly stressed, the body dumps Zinc rapidly.

Good food sources include grass-fed meat, pumpkin seeds, Brazil nuts, broccoli, poultry, oysters, some beans and grains (if they're grown in good soil – and keep in mind, most of our food is produced in depleted soil). Vegetarians, chronic dieters, the elderly, and people who subsist mostly on grains are at particular risk for Zinc deficiency. As a supplement, you should consume no more than 25 mg to 30 mg of Zinc Picolinate (the best absorbed form) every few days, unless a qualified health practitioner recommends taking a higher dose (50 mg to 100 mg/day).

RESOURCES

Eating Disorders

- Academy for Eating Disorders: www.aedweb.org
- Association for Size Diversity and Health – Health at Every Size: www.sizediversityandhealth.org
- Beyond Hunger: www.BeyondHunger.org
- Binge Eating Disorders Association (BEDA): www.bedaonline.com
- National Eating Disorders Association (NEDA): www.nationaleatingdisorders.org
- National Institute of Mental Health, Eating Disorders: www.nimh.nih.gov/health/publications/eating-disorders
- Rosenfeld, S.M., Ph.D.: *Does Every Woman Have an Eating Disorder? Challenging Our Nation's Fixation with Food and Weight*
- Geneen Roth, eating disorders coach: www.GeneenRoth.com

Hospital-Based PCOS Programs

- Brigham and Women's Hospital: www.brighamandwomens.org
- Johns Hopkins Medicine: www.hopkinsmedicine.org
- University of California, San Francisco: www.ucsf.edu

Medical Doctors and Naturopaths

- American Association of Naturopathic Physicians: www. naturopathic.org
- Briden, Lara, ND: *The Period Repair Manual*: www.LaraBriden.com
- Futterweit, W., MD: *A Patient's Guide to PCOS*
- Gersh, Felice, MD: www.felicelgershmd.com
- Gilbert, C.E., MD, PhD: *Dr. Chris's A, B, C's of Health: When Your Body Screams, Listen to It!*
- Gottfried, Sara, MD: *The Hormone Cure: Reclaim Balance, Sleep, Sex Drive & Vitality Naturally with The Gottfried Protocol*
- Harwin, Rebecca, DC: *Conquer Your PCOS Naturally*, www. conqueryourPCOSnaturally.com
- McCulloch, Fiona, ND: *8 Steps to Reverse Your PCOS*, www. drfionand.com
- Moore, Lisa, MD: (310) 829-4528
- Najmabadi, Sam, MD: Center For Reproductive Health & Gynecology, www.reproductive.org
- Cohan, Pejman, MD: (310) 657-3030
- Perloe, Marc, MD: www.arcfertility.com
- Peters, Anne L., MD: *Conquering Diabetes: A Complete Program for Prevention and Treatment*
- Reinholtz, Katie, ND: www.willowbankwellness.com
- Sherif, Katherine, MD: Jefferson University Hospitals, https:// hospitals.jefferson.edu/departments-and-services/womens-primary-care.html

Mental Health

- American Board of Integrative and Holistic Medicine (search for physicians board-certified in holistic and integrative medicine, including psychiatrists): www.abihm.org
- Burns, David D, MD: *The Feeling Good Handbook*

- Cass, Hyla, MD, and Holford, Patrick: *Natural Highs: Supplements, Nutrition, and Mind-Body Techniques to Help You Feel Good All the Time*
- Green Mountain at Fox Run (PCOS-savvy retreat): www.fitwoman.com
- Kubacky, Gretchen, Psy.D., The PCOS Psychologist: www.PCOSwellness.com, www.DrGretchenKubacky.com
- National Alliance on Mental Illness: www.nami.org
- National Suicide Prevention Hotline, USA: (800) 273-8255
- Wiley, T.S. with Formby, B., Ph.D.: *Lights Out: Sleep, Sugar, and Survival*

Mindfulness/Meditation/Buddhist Psychology

- Alexander, Ronald A., Ph.D.: *Wise Mind/Open Mind: Finding Purpose and Meaning in Times of Crisis, Loss & Change*
- Benson, H., M.D.: *The Relaxation Response*
- Bodhipaksa: *Guided Meditation for Calmness, Awareness and Love* (CD)
- Brach, T., Ph.D.: *Radical Acceptance: Embracing Your Life with the Heart of a Buddha*
- Chodron, P.: *When Things Fall Apart*
- Kabat-Zinn, J.: *Guided Mindfulness Meditation – Series 1* (CD)
- Kabat-Zinn, J.: *Wherever You Go, There You Are: Mindfulness Meditation in Everyday Life*
- Reilly, J.L., Ph.D.: *Progressive Deep Muscle Relaxation*
- Siegel, B.: *Meditation for Peace of Mind*
- **Phone Apps**:
  o Insight Timer
  o Calm
  o Simply Being
  o Headspace
  o iChill
  o Breathe2Relax

o   Simple Habit

o   Pacifica

Nutrition and Fitness Education

- Body Wisdom Media: *Yoga for Beginners*
- Cattaneo, Stefania, MS, RDN, Pharm.D.: www.lotusflowerPCOS. com/en
- Dillon, Julie Duffy, RD: www.juliedillonrd.com
- Dopart, Susan, MS, RD, CDE: <u>www.SusanDopart.com</u>
- www.Gaiam.com: *AM/PM Yoga, Rodney Yee's Yoga for Beginners*
- Grassi, Angela, MS, RD, LDN: PCOS Nutrition Center, *The PCOS Workbook: Your Guide to Complete Physical and Emotional Health,* <u>www.pcosnutrition.com</u>
- McKittrick, Martha, MS, RD, CDE: www.marthamckittrick nutrition.com
- Medling, Amy: *Healing PCOS: A 21-Day Plan for Reclaiming Your Health and Life with Polycystic Ovary Syndrome,* www.PCOSdiva. com
- My Fitness Pal, <u>www.MyFitnessPal.com</u>
- Prepon, Laura & Troy, E: *The Stash Plan: Your 21-Day Guide to Shed Weight, Feel Great, and Take Charge of Your Health,* www. thestashplan.com
- Recitas, Lyn-Genet, *The Metabolism Plan: Discover the Foods and Exercises that Work for Your Body to Reduce Inflammation and Drop Pounds Fast*
- Scott, Trudy, CN: www.everywomanover29.com
- Volk, Erika, PCOS Personal Trainer: www.erikavolkfitness.com
- Wright, Hillary, M.Ed., RDN: *The PCOS Diet Plan: A Natural Approach to Health for Women with Polycystic Ovary Syndrome (Second Edition)*

Organizations

- American Society for Reproductive Medicine: www.ASRM.org
- Androgen Excess and PCOS Society: www.ae-society.org
- Jean Hailes for Women's Health: https://jeanhailes.org.au/health-a-z/pcos/weight
- PCOS Awareness Association: www.PCOSAA.org
- PCOS Challenge: The Support System to Help Women Beat PCOS www.PCOSchallenge.org
- PCOS Foundation: www.pcosfoundation.org
- PCOS Wellness: www.PCOSwellness.com
- Polycystic Ovary Association: www.pcosupport.org
- Polycystic Ovary Syndrome Association of Australia: https://www.facebook.com/PCOSAustralia
- RESOLVE: The National Infertility Association: www.resolve.org
- Soul Cysters: www.soulcysters.com
- Verity: www.verity-pcos.org.uk

References

Chapter 1: What is PCOS?

DuRant, E., & Leslie, N. S. (2007). Polycystic Ovary Syndrome: A Review of Current Knowledge. *The Journal for Nurse Practitioners, 3*(3), 180–185. http://doi.org/https://doi.org/10.1016/j.nurpra.2007.01.018

Greco, T., Graham, C. A., Bancroft, J., Tanner, A., & Doll, H. A. (2007). The effects of oral contraceptives on androgen levels and their relevance to premenstrual mood and sexual interest: a comparison of two triphasic formulations containing norgestimate and either 35 or 25 g of ethinyl estradiol. *Contraception, 76*(1), 8–17. http://doi.org/10.1016/j.contraception.2007.04.002

Azziz, R. (2006). Diagnosis of Polycystic Ovarian Syndrome: The Rotterdam Criteria Are Premature. *The Journal of Clinical Endocrinology & Metabolism, 91*(3), 781–785. Retrieved from http://dx.doi.org/10.1210/jc.2005-2153

Fauser, B. C. J. M. (2004). Revised 2003 consensus on diagnostic criteria and long-term health risks related to polycystic ovary syndrome. *Fertility and Sterility, 81*(1), 19–25. http://doi.org/10.1016/j.fertnstert.2003.10.004

Teede, H., Deeks, A., & Moran, L. (2010). Polycystic ovary syndrome: a complex condition with psychological, reproductive and metabolic manifestations that impacts on health across the lifespan. *BMC Medicine, 8,* 41. http://doi.org/10.1186/1741-7015-8-41

Hall, M. F., & Hall, S. E. (2017). *Managing the psychological impact of medical trauma: A guide for mental health and health care professionals.* New York, NY, US: Springer Publishing Co.

Chapter 3: Hormones, Mood, and Stress

Woolsey M., What is PCOS? The Perfect Endocrine Storm Enewsletter. March 2006. Available at http://www.afterthediet.com/polycyst2.html. Accessed May 8, 2006.

Lupien, S. J., McEwen, B. S., Gunnar, M. R., & Heim, C. (2009). Effects of stress throughout the lifespan on the brain, behaviour and cognition. *Nat Rev Neurosci, 10*(6), 434–445. Retrieved from http://dx.doi.org/10.1038/nrn2639

Davis, S. R., & Tran, J. (2001). Testosterone influences libido and well being in women. *Trends in Endocrinology & Metabolism, 12*(1), 33–37. http://doi.org/10.1016/S1043-2760(00)00333-7

Shapiro, S. (2001). Addressing postmenopausal estrogen deficiency: a position paper of the American Council on Science and Health. *MedGenMed : Medscape General Medicine.* Obstetrics and Gynecology, Women's Endocrine Services, Reproductive Endocrinology-Physiology Program, University of Wisconsin, Madison, USA. Retrieved from http://europepmc.org/abstract/MED/11320346

Varney, N. R., Syrop, C., Kubu, C. S., Struchen, M., Hahn, S., & Franzen, K. (1993). Neuropsychologic dysfunction in women following leuprolide acetate induction of hypoestrogenism. *Journal of Assisted Reproduction and Genetics, 10*(1), 53–57. http://doi.org/10.1007/BF01204441

Lokuge, S., Frey, B. N., Foster, J. A., Soares, C. N., & Steiner, M. (2011). Depression in women: windows of vulnerability and new insights into the link between estrogen and serotonin. *The Journal of Clinical Psychiatry, 72*(11), e1563-9. http://doi.org/10.4088/jcp.11com07089

Janssen, O. E., Mehlmauer, N., Hahn, S., Offner, A. H., & Gärtner, R. (2004). High prevalence of autoimmune thyroiditis in patients with polycystic ovary syndrome. *European Journal of Endocrinology / European*

Federation of Endocrine Societies, 150(3), 363–9. http://doi.org/10.1530/eje.0.1500363

Shealy, C. N. (1995). A review of dehydroepiandrosterone (DHEA). *Integrative Physiological and Behavioral Science, 30*(4), 308–313. http://doi.org/10.1007/BF02691603

Michael, A., Jenaway, A., Paykel, E. S., & Herbert, J. (2000). Altered Salivary Dehydroepiandrosterone Levels in Major Depression in Adults. *Biological Psychiatry,* (48), 989–995. Retrieved from https://pdfs.semanticscholar.org/14d6/ee4585285a47e47586323ab0449530014969.pdf

Thompson, C., Stinson, D., & Smith, A. (1990). Seasonal affective disorder and season-dependent abnormalities of melatonin suppression by light. *The Lancet, 336*(8717), 703–706. http://doi.org/http://dx.doi.org/10.1016/0140-6736(90)92202-S

Hardeland, R. (2012). Neurobiology, Pathophysiology, and Treatment of Melatonin Deficiency and Dysfunction. *The Scientific World Journal, 2012*, 1–18. http://doi.org/10.1100/2012/640389

Seida, J. C., Mitri, J., Colmers, I. N., Majumdar, S. R., Davidson, M. B., Edwards, A. L., ... Johnson, J. A. (2014). Effect of Vitamin D(3) Supplementation on Improving Glucose Homeostasis and Preventing Diabetes: A Systematic Review and Meta-Analysis. *The Journal of Clinical Endocrinology and Metabolism, 99*(10), 3551–3560. http://doi.org/10.1210/jc.2014-2136

Gominak, S. C., & Stumpf, W. E. (2012). The world epidemic of sleep disorders is linked to vitamin D deficiency. *Medical Hypotheses, 79*(2), 132–135. http://doi.org/http://dx.doi.org/10.1016/j.mehy.2012.03.031

Berk, M., Berk, M., Sanders, K. M., Pasco, J. A., Jacka, F. N., Williams, L. J., ... Dodd, S. (2014). Vitamin D deficiency may play a role in depression, (February), 1–5. http://doi.org/10.1016/j.mehy.2007.04.001

Chapters 5: Insomnia and Other Sleep Disorders and 17: Improving Sleep

Hirshkowitz, M., Whiton, K., Albert, S. M., Alessi, C., Bruni, O., DonCarlos, L., ... Adams Hillard, P. J. (2015). National sleep foundation's sleep time duration recommendations: Methodology and results summary. *Sleep Health*, 1(1), 40–43. http://doi.org/10.1016/j.sleh.2014.12.010

Ferrara, M., & De Gennaro, L. (2001). How much sleep do we need? *Sleep Medicine Reviews*, 5(2), 155–179. http://doi.org/10.1053/smrv.2000.0138

Ehrmann, D. A. (2012). Metabolic dysfunction in PCOS: Relationship to obstructive sleep apnea. *Steroids*, 77(4), 290–294. http://doi.org/10.1016/j.steroids.2011.12.001

Kahn-Greene, E. T., Killgore, D. B., Kamimori, G. H., Balkin, T. J., & Killgore, W. D. S. (2007). The effects of sleep deprivation on symptoms of psychopathology in healthy adults. *Sleep Medicine*, 8(3), 215–221. http://doi.org/10.1016/j.sleep.2006.08.007

American Psychiatric Association. (2013). *Diagnostic and statistical manual of mental disorders (DSM-5®)*. American Psychiatric Pub.

Franik, G., Krysta, K., Madej, P., Gimlewicz-Pieta, B., Oslizlo, B., Trukawka, J., & Olszanecka-Glinianowicz, M. (2016). Sleep disturbances in women with polycystic ovary syndrome. *Gynecological Endocrinology : The Official Journal of the International Society of Gynecological Endocrinology*, 3590 (September 2016), 1–4. http://doi.org/10.1080/09513590.2016.1196177

Punjabi, N. M. (2008). The epidemiology of adult obstructive sleep apnea. *Proceedings of the American Thoracic Society*, 5(2), 136–43. http://doi.org/10.1513/pats.200709-155MG

Ayas, N. T., White, D. P., Manson, J. E., Stampfer, M. J., Speizer, F. E., Malhotra, A., & Hu, F. B. (2003). A Prospective Study of Sleep Duration and Coronary Heart Disease in Women. *Archives of Internal Medicine*, 163(2), 205. http://doi.org/10.1001/archinte.163.2.205

Shahar, E., Whitney, C. W., Redline, S., Lee, E. T., Newman, A. B., Javler, F., ... Samet, J. M. (2001). Sleep-disordered breathing and cardiovascular disease: Cross-sectional results of the sleep heart health study. *American Journal of Respiratory and Critical Care Medicine, 163*(1), 19–25. http://doi.org/10.1164/ajrccm.163.1.2001008

Snel, J., & Lorist, M. M. (2011). *Effects of caffeine on sleep and cognition. Progress in Brain Research* (1st ed., Vol. 190). Elsevier B.V. http://doi.org/10.1016/B978-0-444-53817-8.00006-2

Tasali, E., Cauter, E. Van, & Ehrmann, D. (2008). Polycystic Ovary Syndrom and Obstructive Sleep Apnea. *Sleep Medicine Clinics, 3*(1), 37–46. Retrieved from http://www.sciencedirect.com/science/article/pii/S1556407X07001415

Chakraborty, P., Ghosh, S., Goswami, S. K., Kabir, S. N., Chakravarty, B., & Jana, K. (2013). Altered trace mineral milieu might play an aetiological role in the pathogenesis of polycystic ovary syndrome. *Biological Trace Element Research, 152*(1), 9–15. http://doi.org/10.1007/s12011-012-9592-5

El-Serag, H. B., Ergun, G. A., Pandolfino, J., Fitzgerald, S., Tran, T., & Kramer, J. R. (2007). Obesity increases oesophageal acid exposure. *Gut, 56*(6), 749–755. http://doi.org/10.1136/gut.2006.100263

Mannel, M. (2004). Drug Interactions with St John's Wort. *Drug Safety, 27*(11), 773–797. http://doi.org/10.2165/00002018-200427110-00003

Chapter 10: Prescription Medications, Foods, and Procedures

(2015). *Medicines Use and Spending Shifts: A Review of the Use of Medicines in the U.S. in 2014.* IMS Institute for Healthcare Informatics. Retrieved on 8/12/17 from: http://www.imshealth.com/en/thought-leadership/quintilesims-institute/reports/medicines-use-in-the-us-2014#ims-form

(July 8, 2015). *Multivitamin/mineral Supplements: Fact Sheet for Health Professionals.* National Institutes of Health, Office of Dietary Supplements. Retrieved from: https://ods.od.nih.gov/factsheets/MVMS-HealthProfessional/#en3

Chapter 11: Selective Supplementation and Other Tools

Bhattacharya, S. M., & Jha, A. (2010). Prevalence and risk of depressive disorders in women with polycystic ovary syndrome (PCOS). Fertility and Sterility, 94(1), 357–359. http://doi.org/10.1016/j.fertnstert.2009.09.025

Barry, J. A., Kuczmierczyk, A. R., & Hardiman, P. J. (2011). Anxiety and depression in polycystic ovary syndrome: A systematic review and meta-analysis. Human Reproduction, 26(9), 2442–2451. http://doi.org/10.1093/humrep/der197

Fogel, R. B., Malhotra, A., Pillar, G., Pittman, S. D., Dunaif, a, & White, D. P. (2001). Increased prevalence of obstructive sleep apnea syndrome in obese women with polycystic ovary syndrome. The Journal of Clinical Endocrinology and Metabolism, 86(3), 1175–1180. http://doi.org/10.1210/jcem.86.3.7316

Masharani, U., Gjerde, C., Evans, J. L., Youngren, J. F., & Goldfine, I. D. (2010). Effects of Controlled-Release Alpha Lipoic Acid in Lean, Nondiabetic Patients with Polycystic Ovary Syndrome. Journal of Diabetes Science and Technology, 4(2), 359–364. http://doi.org/10.1177/193229681000400218

Stevens, M. J., Obrosova, I., Cao, X., Van Huysen, C., & Greene, D. A. (2000). Effects of DL-α-Lipoic Acid on Peripheral Nerve Conduction, Blood Flow, Energy Metabolism, and Oxidative Stress in Experimental Diabetic Neuropathy. Diabetes, 49, 1006–1015.

Cappelli, V., Di Sabatino, A., Musacchio, M. C., & De Leo, V. (2013). [Evaluation of a new association between insulin-sensitizers and α-lipoic acid in obese women affected by PCOS]. Minerva ginecologica, 65(4), 425–433. Retrieved from http://europepmc.org/abstract/MED/24051942

Jiang, T., Yin, F., Yao, J., Brinton, R. D., & Cadenas, E. (2013). Lipoic acid restores age-associated impairment of brain energy metabolism through the modulation of Akt/JNK signaling and PGC1α transcriptional pathway. Aging Cell, 12(6), 1021–1031. http://doi.org/10.1111/acel.12127

Packer, L., Witt, E. H., & Tritschler, H. J. (1995). Alpha-lipoic acid as a biological antioxidant. Free Radical Biology and Medicine, 19(2), 227–250. http://doi.org/10.1016/0891-5849(95)00017-R

Pratte, M. A., Nanavati, K. B., Young, V., & Morley, C. P. (2014). An alternative treatment for anxiety: a systematic review of human trial results reported for the Ayurvedic herb ashwagandha (Withania somnifera). *Journal of Alternative and Complementary Medicine, 20*(12), 901–8. http://doi.org/10.1089/acm.2014.0177

Verma, S. K., & Kumar, A. (2011). THERAPEUTIC USES OF WITHANIA SOMNIFERA (ASHWAGANDHA) WITH A NOTE ON WITHANOLIDES AND ITS PHARMACOLOGICAL ACTIONS. *Asian Journal of Pharmaceutical and Clinical Research, 4*(Suppl 1), 1–4.

Parletta, N., Milte, C. M., & Meyer, B. J. (2013). Nutritional modulation of cognitive function and mental health. *Journal of Nutritional Biochemistry, 24*(5), 725–743. http://doi.org/10.1016/j.jnutbio.2013.01.002

Sun, Y., Lai, M.-S., & Lu, C.-J. (2005). Effectiveness of vitamin B12 on diabetic neuropathy: systematic review of clinical controlled trials. *Acta Neurologica Taiwanica, 14*(2), 48–54.

Andrès, E., Loukili, N. H., Noel, E., Kaltenbach, G., Ben Abdelgheni, M., Perrin, A. E., … Blicklé, J. F. (2004). Vitamin B12 (cobalamin) deficiency in elderly patients. *Cmaj, 171*(3), 251–259. http://doi.org/10.1503/cmaj.1031155

Alpert, J. E., & Fava, M. (1997). Nutrition and depression: the role of folate. *Nutrition Reviews, 55*(5), 145–149. http://doi.org/10.1111/j.1753-4887.1997.tb06468.x

Reinstatler, L., Qi, Y. P., Williamson, R. S., Garn, J. V., & Oakley, G. P. (2012). Association of biochemical B 12 deficiency with metformin therapy and vitamin B 12 supplements: The National Health and Nutrition Examination Survey, 1999-2006. *Diabetes Care, 35*(2), 327–333. http://doi.org/10.2337/dc11-1582

Zhang, J., Tang, H., Deng, R., Wang, N., Zhang, Y., Wang, Y., … Zhou, L. (2015). Berberine suppresses adipocyte differentiation via decreasing CREB transcriptional activity. *PLoS ONE, 10*(4), 1–16. http://doi.org/10.1371/journal.pone.0125667

Cerda, C., Pérez-Ayuso, R. M., Riquelme, A., Soza, A., Villaseca, P., Sir-Petermann, T., … Arrese, M. (2007). Nonalcoholic fatty liver disease in women with polycystic ovary syndrome. *Journal of Hepatology, 47*(3), 412–417. http://doi.org/10.1016/j.jhep.2007.04.012

Li, Z., Geng, Y.-N., Jiang, J.-D., & Kong, W.-J. (2014). Antioxidant and anti-inflammatory activities of berberine in the treatment of diabetes mellitus. *Evidence-Based Complementary and Alternative Medicine: eCAM, 2014*, 289264. http://doi.org/10.1155/2014/289264

EFSA Panel on Dietetic Products, N. and A. (NDA). (2010). Scientific Opinion on the substantiation of health claims related to biotin and maintenance of normal skin and mucous membranes (ID 121), maintenance of normal hair (ID 121), maintenance of normal bone (ID 121), maintenance of normal teeth (ID 121. *EFSA Journal, 8*(10), 1–19. http://doi.org/10.2903/j.efsa.2010.1728.

Furukawa, Y. (1999). [Enhancement of glucose-induced insulin secretion and modification of glucose metabolism by biotin]. *Nihon rinsho. Japanese journal of clinical medicine, 57*(10), 2261–2269. Retrieved from http://europepmc.org/abstract/MED/10540872

Koutsikos, D., Agroyannis, B., & Tzanatos-Exarchou, H. (1990). Biotin for diabetic peripheral neuropathy. *Biomedicine & Pharmacotherapy, 44*(10), 511–514. http://doi.org/http://dx.doi.org/10.1016/0753-3322(90)90171-5

Albarracin, C. A., Fuqua, B. C., Evans, J. L., & Goldfine, I. D. (2008). Chromium picolinate and biotin combination improves glucose metabolism in treated, uncontrolled overweight to obese patients with type 2 diabetes. *Diabetes/Metabolism Research and Reviews, 24*(1), 41–51. http://doi.org/10.1002/dmrr.755

Healy, D. L., Trounson, A. O., & Andersen, A. N. (1994). Female infertility: causes and treatment. *The Lancet, 343*(8912), 1539–1544. http://doi.org/http://dx.doi.org/10.1016/S0140-6736(94)92941-6

Irvine, D. S. (1998). Epidemiology and aetiology of male infertility. *Human Reproduction, 13*(Supplement 1), 33–44.

Bremer, J. (1983). Carnitine–metabolism and functions. *Physiological Reviews, 63*(4), 1420–1480. Retrieved from http://www.ncbi.nlm.nih.gov/pubmed/6361812

Singletary, K. (2008). Cinnamon: Overview of health benefits. *Nutrition Today, 43*(6), 263–266. http://doi.org/10.1097/01.NT.0000342702.19798.fe

Hlebowicz, J., Darwiche, G., Björgell, O., & Almér, L. O. (2007). Effect of cinnamon on postprandial blood glucose, gastric emptying, and satiety in healthy subjects. *American Journal of Clinical Nutrition, 85*(6), 1552–1556. http://doi.org/10.1186/1475-2891-8-26

Sarter, B. (2002). Coenzyme Q10 and Cardiovascular Disease: A Review. *Journal of Cardiovascular Nursing, 16*(4). Retrieved from http://journals.lww.com/jcnjournal/Fulltext/2002/07000/Coenzyme_Q10_and_Cardiovascular_Disease__A_Review.3.aspx

Anderson, R. A., Cheng, N., Bryden, N. A., Polansky, M. M., Cheng, N., Chi, J., & Feng, J. (1997). Elevated Intakes of Supplemental Chromium Improve Glucose and Insulin Variables in Individuals With Type 2 Diabetes. *Diabetes, 46*(11), 1786 LP-1791. Retrieved from http://diabetes.diabetesjournals.org/content/46/11/1786.abstract

Lydic, M. L., McNurlan, M., Komaroff, E., Mitchell, L., Bembo, S., & Gelato, M. (2003). Effects of chromium supplementation on insulin sensitivity and reproductive function in polycystic ovarian syndrome: A pilot study. *Fertility and Sterility, 80,* 45-46.

Gilbody, S., Lewis, S., & Lightfoot, T. (2007). Methylenetetrahydrofolate reductase (MTHFR) genetic polymorphisms and psychiatric disorders: A HuGE review. *American Journal of Epidemiology, 165*(1), 1–13. http://doi.org/10.1093/aje/kwj347

Fava, M., & Mischoulon, D. (2009). Folate in depression: Efficacy, safety, differences in formulations, and clinical issues. *Journal of Clinical Psychiatry, 70*(SUPPL. 5), 12–17. http://doi.org/10.4088/JCP.8157su1c.03

Schmidt, P. J., Daly, R. C., Bloch, M., Smith, M. J., Danaceau, M. a, St Clair, L. S., ... Rubinow, D. R. (2005). Dehydroepiandrosterone monotherapy in midlife-onset major and minor depression. *Archives of General Psychiatry, 62*(2), 154–62. http://doi.org/10.1001/archpsyc.62.2.154

Buoso, E., Lanni, C., Molteni, E., Rousset, F., Corsini, E., & Racchi, M. (2011). Opposing effects of cortisol and dehydroepiandrosterone on the expression of the receptor for Activated C Kinase 1: Implications in immunosenescence. *Experimental Gerontology, 46*(11), 877–883. http://doi.org/10.1016/j.exger.2011.07.007

Azziz, R., Carmina, E., Dewailly, D., Diamanti-Kandarakis, E., Escobar-Morreale, H. F., Futterweit, W., ... Witchel, S. F. (2009). *The Androgen Excess and PCOS Society criteria for the polycystic ovary syndrome:*

the complete task force report. *Fertility and Sterility* (Vol. 91). http://doi.org/10.1016/j.fertnstert.2008.06.035

Nair, K. S., Rizza, R. A., O'Brien, P., Dhatariya, K., Short, K. R., Nehra, A., ... Jensen, M. D. (2006). DHEA in elderly women and DHEA or testosterone in elderly men. *The New England Journal of Medicine*, 355(16), 1647–59. http://doi.org/10.1056/NEJMoa054629

Alkatib, A. a, Cosma, M., Elamin, M. B., Erickson, D., Swiglo, B. a, Erwin, P. J., & Montori, V. M. (2009). A systematic review and meta-analysis of randomized placebo-controlled trials of DHEA treatment effects on quality of life in women with adrenal insufficiency. *The Journal of Clinical Endocrinology and Metabolism*, 94(10), 3676–3681. http://doi.org/10.1210/jc.2009-0672

Kravitz, H. M., Sabelli, H. C., & Fawcett, J. (1984). Dietary supplements of phenylalanine and other amino acid precursors of brain neuroamines in the treatment of depressive disorders. *Journal of the American Osteopathic Association*, 84(1 SUPPL.), 119-123.

Fux, M., Levine, J., Aviv, A., & Belmaker, R. H. (1996). Inositol treatment of obsessive-compulsive disorder. *American Journal of Psychiatry*, 153(9), 1219–1221. http://doi.org/10.1176/ajp.153.9.1219

J., B., J., L., M., F., A., A., D., L., & R.H., B. (1995). Double-blind, placebo-controlled, crossover trial of inositol treatment for panic disorder. *American Journal of Psychiatry*, 152(7), 1084–1086. http://doi.org/10.1176/ajp.152.7.1084

Abdelhamid, A. M. S., Ismail Madkour, W. A., & Borg, T. F. (2015). Inositol versus metformin administration in polycystic ovarian disease patients. *Evidence Based Women's Health Journal*, 5(2), 61–66. http://doi.org/10.1097/01.EBX.0000462483.99152.8d

Cerda, C., Pérez-Ayuso, R. M., Riquelme, A., Soza, A., Villaseca, P., Sir-Petermann, T., ... Arrese, M. (2007). Nonalcoholic fatty liver disease in women with polycystic ovary syndrome. *Journal of Hepatology*, 47(3), 412–417. http://doi.org/10.1016/j.jhep.2007.04.012

Costantino, D., Minozzi, G., Minozzi, E., & Guaraldi, C. (2009). Metabolic and hormonal effects of myo-inositol in women with polycystic ovary syndrome: a double-blind trial. *European Review for Medical and*

Pharmacological Sciences, *13*, 105–10. Retrieved from http://www.ncbi.nlm.nih.gov/pubmed/19499845

Nestler, J. E., & Unfer, V. (2015). Reflections on inositol(s) for PCOS therapy: steps toward success. *Gynecological Endocrinology: The Official Journal of the International Society of Gynecological Endocrinology*, *31*(7), 501–5. http://doi.org/10.3109/09513590.2015.1054802

Hirata, J. D., Small, R., Swiersz, L. M., Ettinger, B., & Zell, B. (1997). Does dong quai have estrogenic effects in postmenopausal women? A double-blind, placebo-controlled trial. *Fertility and Sterility*, *68*(6), 981–986. http://doi.org/10.1016/S0015-0282(97)00397-X

Hardy, M. (2000). Herbs of Special Interest to Women. *J Am Pharm Assoc*, *40*(2), 234–242. http://doi.org/10.1016/S1086-5802(16)31064-6

L. Kunkel, S., Ogawa, H., A. Ward, P., & B. Zurier, R. (1981). Suppression of chronic inflammation by evening primrose oil. *Progress in Lipid Research*, *20*, 885–888. http://doi.org/http://dx.doi.org/10.1016/0163-7827(81)90165-X

Belch, J. J. F., & Hill, A. (2000). Evening primrose oil and borage oil in rheumatologic conditions. *American Journal of Clinical Nutrition*, *71*(1 SUPPL.), 352–356.

BYERLEY, W. F., JUDD, L. L., REIMHERR, F. W., & GROSSER, B. I. (1987). 5-Hydroxytryptophan: A Review of Its Antidepressant Efficacy and Adverse Effects. *Journal of Clinical Psychopharmacology*, *7*(3). Retrieved from http://journals.lww.com/psychopharmacology/Fulltext/1987/06000/5_Hydroxytryptophan___A_Review_of_Its.2.aspx

Ravindran, A. V., & Da Silva, T. L. (2013). Complementary and alternative therapies as add-on to pharmacotherapy for mood and anxiety disorders: A systematic review. *Journal of Affective Disorders*, *150*(3), 707–719. http://doi.org/10.1016/j.jad.2013.05.042

Diana, M., Quilez, J., & Rafecas, M. (2014). Gamma-aminobutyric acid as a bioactive compound in foods: A review. *Journal of Functional Foods*, (10), 407–420

Aggarwal, B., & Harikumar, K. (2009). Potential Therapeutic Effects of Curcumin, the Anti-inflammatory Agent, Against Neurodegenerative, Cardiovascular, Pulmonary, Metabolic, Autoimmune and Neoplastic

Diseases Bharat. *International Journal of Biochemistry and Cell Biology,* *41*(1), 40–59. http://doi.org/10.1016/j.biocel.2008.06.010.

Akinyemi, A. J., Thome, G. R., Morsch, V. M., Stefanello, N., da Costa, P., Cardoso, A., ... Schetinger, M. R. C. (2016). Effect of dietary supplementation of ginger and turmeric rhizomes on ectonucleotidases, adenosine deaminase and acetylcholinesterase activities in synaptosomes from the cerebral cortex of hypertensive rats. *Journal of Applied Biomedicine,* *14*(1), 59–70. http://doi.org/http://dx.doi.org/10.1016/j.jab.2015.06.001

Singletary, K. (2010). Ginger: An Overview of Health Benefits. *Nutrition Today, 45*(4), 171–183. http://doi.org/10.1097/NT.0b013e3181ed3543

Vélez, L. M., & Motta, A. B. (2014). Association between polycystic ovary syndrome and metabolic syndrome. *Current Medicinal Chemistry,* *21*(35), 3999–4012. http://doi.org/10.2174/09298673216661409151410 30

Shanmugasundaram, E. R. B., Rajeswari, G., Baskaran, K., Kumar, B. R. R., Shanmugasundaram, K. R., & Ahmath, B. K. (1990). Use of Gymnema sylvestre leaf extract in the control of blood glucose in insulin-dependent diabetes mellitus. *Journal of Ethnopharmacology, 30*(3), 281–294. http://doi.org/http://dx.doi.org/10.1016/0378-8741(90)90107-5

Sarris, J. (2010). An explorative qualitative analysis of participants' experience of using kava versus placebo in an RCT. *Australian Journal of Medical Herbalism, 22*(1), 12–16. Retrieved from www.ebscohost.com

Russo, M. W., Galanko, J. A., Shrestha, R., Fried, M. W., & Watkins, P. (2004). Liver transplantation for acute liver failure from drug induced liver injury in the United States. *Liver Transplantation, 10*(8), 1018–1023. http://doi.org/10.1002/lt.20204

Cavanagh, H. M. A., & Wilkinson, J. M. (2002). Biological activities of lavender essential oil. *Phytotherapy Research, 16*(4), 301–308. http://doi.org/10.1002/ptr.1103

Even, C., Schröder, C. M., Friedman, S., & Rouillon, F. (2008). Efficacy of light therapy in nonseasonal depression: A systematic review. *Journal of Affective Disorders, 108*(1–2), 11–23. http://doi.org/10.1016/j.jad.2007.09.008

Sit, D., Wisner, K. L., Hanusa, B. H., Stull, S., & Terman, M. (2007).

Light therapy for bipolar disorder: A case series in women. *Bipolar Disorders*, 9(8), 918–927. http://doi.org/10.1111/j.1399-5618.2007.00451.x

Déchelotte, P., Hasselmann, M., Cynober, L., Allaouchiche, B., Coëffier, M., Hecketsweiler, B., ... Bleichner, G. (2006). L-alanyl-L-glutamine dipeptide-supplemented total parenteral nutrition reduces infectious complications and glucose intolerance in critically ill patients: the French controlled, randomized, double-blind, multicenter study. *Critical Care Medicine*, 34(3), 598–604. http://doi.org/10.1097/01. CCM.0000201004.30750.D1

Miller, A. L. (1999). Therapeutic considerations of L-glutamine: a review of the literature. *Alternative Medicine Review: A Journal of Clinical Therapeutic*, 4(4), 239–248. Retrieved from http://europepmc.org/ abstract/MED/10468648

Goyal, M., Singh, S., Sibinga, E. M. S., Gould, N. F., Rowland-Seymour, A., Sharma, R., ... Haythornthwaite, J. A. (2014). Meditation Programs for Psychological Stress and Well-being. *JAMA Internal Medicine*, 174(3), 357. http://doi.org/10.1001/jamainternmed.2013.13018

Geddes, J. R., Burgess, S., Hawton, K., Jamison, K., & Goodwin, G. M. (2004). Long-Term Lithium Therapy for Bipolar Disorder: Systematic Review and Meta-Analysis of Randomized Controlled Trials. *American Journal of Psychiatry*, 161(2), 217–222. http://doi.org/10.1176/appi. ajp.161.2.217

Chiu, C.-T., Wang, Z., Hunsberger, J. G., & Chuang, D.-M. (2013). Therapeutic Potential of Mood Stabilizers Lithium and Valproic Acid: Beyond Bipolar Disorder. *Pharmacological Reviews*, 65(1), 105–142. http://doi.org/10.1124/pr.111.005512

Vita, A., De Peri, L., & Sacchetti, E. (2015). Lithium in drinking water and suicide prevention. *International Clinical Psychopharmacology*, 30(1), 1–5. http://doi.org/10.1097/YIC.0000000000000048

Schrauzer, G. N., & Shrestha, K. P. (1990). Lithium in drinking water and the incidences of crimes, suicides, and arrests related to drug addictions. *Biological Trace Element Research*, 25(2), 105–113. http://doi. org/10.1007/BF02990271

Bowden, C. L. (1998). Key treatment studies of lithium in manic-depressive illness: efficacy and side effects. *The Journal of Clinical*

Psychiatry, 59 Suppl 6, 13–9; discussion 20. Retrieved from http://europepmc.org/abstract/MED/9674932

Nobre, A. C., Rao, A., & Owen, G. N. (2008). L-theanine, a natural constituent in tea, and its effect on mental state.: Discovery Service for Endeavour College of Natural Health Library. *Asia Pacific Journal of Clinical Nutrition, 17*(S1), 167–168. Retrieved from http://eds.b.ebscohost.com.ezproxy.endeavour.edu.au/eds/pdfviewer/pdfviewer?sid=8d65ce71-2282-4636-af46-1e40f6e02256%40sessionmgr102&vid=1&hid=114

Nathan, P. J., Kristy Lu, M., & Gray, Oliver, C. (2006). The neuropharmacology of L-theanine (N-ethyl-L-glutamine): A possible neuroprotective and cognitive enhancing agent The Neuropharmacology of L-Theanine (N-Ethyl-L-Glutamine). *Journal of Herbal Pharmacotherupy, 8940*(August 2015), 20–30. http://doi.org/10.1080/J157v06n02

Kimura, K., Ozeki, M., Juneja, L. R., & Ohira, H. (2007). l-Theanine reduces psychological and physiological stress responses. *Biological Psychology, 74*(1), 39–45. http://doi.org/10.1016/j.biopsycho.2006.06.006

Murphy, S. E., Longhitano, C., Ayres, R. E., Cowen, P. J., & Harmer, C. J. (2006). Tryptophan supplementation induces a positive bias in the processing of emotional material in healthy female volunteers. *Psychopharmacology, 187*(1), 121–130. http://doi.org/10.1007/s00213-006-0401-8

Young, S. N., & Leyton, M. (2002). The role of serotonin in human mood and social interaction: Insight from altered tryptophan levels. *Pharmacology Biochemistry and Behavior, 71*(4), 857–865. http://doi.org/10.1016/S0091-3057(01)00670-0

Sainio, E. L., Pulkki, K., & Young, S. N. (1996). L-Tryptophan: Biochemical, nutritional and pharmacological aspects. *Amino Acids, 10*(1), 21–47. http://doi.org/10.1007/BF00806091

Boyer, E., & Shannon, M. (2005). The serotonin syndrome. *New England Journal of Medicine.* http://doi.org/10.1056/NEJMra041867

Deijen, J. B., Wientjes, C. J. E., Vullinghs, H. F. M., Cloin, P. A., & Langefeld, J. J. (1999). Tyrosine improves cognitive performance and reduces blood pressure in cadets after one week of a combat training course. *Brain Research Bulletin*, 48(2), 203–209. http://doi.org/10.1016/S0361-9230(98)00163-4

Growdon, J. H., Melamed, E., Logue, M., Hefti, F., & Wurtman, R. J. (1982). Effects of oral L-tyrosine administration on CSF tyrosine and homovallinic acid levels in patients with Parkinson's disease. *Life Sciences*.

Jongkees, B. J., Hommel, B., Kahn, S., & Colzato, L. S. (2015). Effect of tyrosine supplementation on clinical and healthy populations under stress or cognitive demands-A review. *Journal of Psychiatric Research, 70*, 50–57. http://doi.org/10.1016/j.jpsychires.2015.08.014

Higashiura, K., & Shimamoto, K. (2005). [Magnesium and insulin resistance]. *Clinical calcium, 15*(2), 251–254. Retrieved from http://europepmc.org/abstract/MED/15692165

Whang, R. (1987). Magnesium deficiency: Pathogenesis, prevalence, and clinical implications. *The American Journal of Medicine, 82*(3), 24–29. http://doi.org/http://dx.doi.org/10.1016/0002-9343(87)90129-X

Seelig, M. S. (1994). Consequences of magnesium deficiency on the enhancement of stress reactions; preventive and therapeutic implications (a review). *Journal of the American College of Nutrition, 13*(5), 429–446. http://doi.org/10.1080/07315724.1994.10718432

Chakraborty, P., Ghosh, S., Goswami, S. K., Kabir, S. N., Chakravarty, B., & Jana, K. (2013). Altered trace mineral milieu might play an aetiological role in the pathogenesis of polycystic ovary syndrome. *Biological Trace Element Research, 152*(1), 9–15. http://doi.org/10.1007/s12011-012-9592-5

Vélez, L. M., & Motta, A. B. (2014). Association between polycystic ovary syndrome and metabolic syndrome. *Current Medicinal Chemistry, 21*(35), 3999–4012. http://doi.org/10.2174/09298673216661409151430

Guerrero-Romero, F., & Rodríguez-Morán, M. (2002). Low serum magnesium levels and metabolic syndrome. *Acta Diabetologica, 39*(4), 209–213. http://doi.org/10.1007/s005920200036

Wacker, W. E. C., & Parisi, A. F. (1968). Magnesium Metabolism. *New England Journal of Medicine, 278*(12), 658–663. http://doi.org/10.1056/NEJM196803212781205

Shechter, M. (2010). Magnesium and cardiovascular system.

Magnesium Research, 23(2), 60–72. http://doi.org/10.1684/mrh.2010.0202

Lakhan, S. E., & Vieira, K. F. (2010). Nutritional and herbal supplements for anxiety and anxiety-related disorders: systematic review. *Nutrition Journal, 9*, 42. http://doi.org/10.1186/1475-2891-9-42

Hill, K. P. (2015). Medical Marijuana for Treatment of Chronic Pain and Other Medical and Psychiatric Problems. *Jama, 313*(24), 2474. http://doi.org/10.1001/jama.2015.6199

Bergamaschi, M. M., Queiroz, R. H. C., Chagas, M. H. N., de Oliveira, D. C. G., De Martinis, B. S., Kapczinski, F., ... Crippa, J. A. S. (2011). Cannabidiol reduces the anxiety induced by simulated public speaking in treatment-naïve social phobia patients. *Neuropsychopharmacology, 36*(6), 1219–26. http://doi.org/10.1038/npp.2011.6

Zhdanova, I. V., Wurtman, R. J., Lynch, H. J., Ives, J. R., Dollins, A. B., Morabito, C., ... Schomer, D. L. (1995). Sleep-inducing effects of low doses of melatonin ingested in the evening. *Clinical Pharmacology and Therapeutics, 57*(5), 552–558. http://doi.org/10.1016/0009-9236(95)90040-3

Katiyar, S.K. (2005). Silymarin and skin cancer prevention: Anti-inflammatory, antioxidant and immunomodulatory effects (Review). *International Journal of Oncology, 26*, 169-176. https://doi.org/10.3892/ijo.26.1.169

Post-White, J., Ladas, E. J., & Kelly, K. M. (2007). Advances in the use of milk thistle (Silybum marianum). *Integrative Cancer Therapies, 6*(2), 104–109. http://doi.org/10.1177/1534735407301632

Dekhuijzen, P. N. R. (2004). Antioxidant properties of N-acetylcysteine: Their relevance in relation to chronic obstructive pulmonary disease. *European Respiratory Journal, 23*(4), 629–636. http://doi.org/10.1183/09031936.04.00016804

Berk, M., Malhi, G. S., Gray, L. J., & Dean, O. M. (2013). The promise of N-acetylcysteine in neuropsychiatry. *Trends in Pharmacological Sciences, 34*(3), 167–177. http://doi.org/10.1016/j.tips.2013.01.001

Parker, G., Neville Gibson, F. A., Brotchie, H., Gabriella Heruc, B., Rees, A.-M., & Dusan Hadzi-Pavlovic, D. (2006). Omega-3 Fatty Acids and Mood Disorders. *Am J Psychiatry, 1636*(163), 969–978. http://doi.org/10.1176/appi.ajp.163.6.969

Sarris, J., Murphy, J., Mischoulon, D., Papakostas, G. I., Fava, M., Berk, M., & Ng, C. H. (2016). Adjunctive nutraceuticals for depression: A systematic review and meta-analyses. *American Journal of Psychiatry, 173*(6), 575–587. http://doi.org/10.1176/appi.ajp.2016.15091228

Lin, P. Y., & Su, K. P. (2007). A meta-analytic review of double-blind, placebo-controlled trials of antidepressant efficacy of omega-3 fatty acids. *Journal of Clinical Psychiatry, 68*(7), 1056–1061. http://doi.org/10.4088/JCP.v68n0712

Simopoulos, A. P. (2002). The importance of the ratio of omega-6/omega-3 essential fatty acids. *Biomedicine and Pharmacotherapy, 56*(8), 365–379. http://doi.org/10.1016/S0753-3322(02)00253-6

Hawkes, C. (2006). Uneven dietary development: linking the policies and processes of globalization with the nutrition transition, obesity and diet-related chronic diseases. *Globalization and Health, 2*(February), 4. http://doi.org/10.1186/1744-8603-2-4

Blasbalg, T. L., Hibbeln, J. R., Ramsden, C. E., Majchrzak, S. F., & Rawlings, R. R. (2011). Changes in consumption of omega-3 and omega-6 fatty acids in the United States during the 20th century. *American Journal of Clinical Nutrition, 93*(5), 950–962. http://doi.org/10.3945/ajcn.110.006643

Foster, J. A., & McVey Neufeld, K. A. (2013). Gut-brain axis: How the microbiome influences anxiety and depression. *Trends in Neurosciences, 36*(5), 305–312. http://doi.org/10.1016/j.tins.2013.01.005

Vitetta, L., Bambling, M., & Alford, H. (2014). The gastrointestinal tract microbiome, probiotics, and mood. *Inflammopharmacology, 22*(6), 333–339. http://doi.org/10.1007/s10787-014-0216-x

Kelly, G. S. (2001). Rhodiola rosea: A possible plant adaptogen. *Alternative Medicine Review, 6*(3), 293–302.

Bottiglieri, T., Hyland, K., & Reynolds, E. H. (1994). The Clinical Potential of Ademetionine (S-Adenosylmethionine) in Neurological Disorders. *Drugs, 48*(2), 137–152. http://doi.org/10.2165/00003495-199448020-00002

Jacobsen, S., Danneskiold-samsøe, B., & Andersen, R. B. (1991). Oral

S-adenosylmethionine in Primary Fibromyalgia. Double-blind Clinical Evaluation. *Scandinavian Journal of Rheumatology*, 20(4), 294–302. http://doi.org/10.3109/03009749109096803

Soeken, K. L., Lee, W.-L., Bausell, R. B., Agelli, M., & Berman, B. M. (2002). Safety and efficacy of S-adenosylmethionine (SAMe) for osteoarthritis. *The Journal of Family Practice*, 51(5), 425–30. http://doi.org/jfp_0502_00425 [pii]

Sarris, J., Murphy, J., Mischoulon, D., Papakostas, G. I., Fava, M., Berk M., & Ng, C. H. (2016). Adjunctive nutraceuticals for depression: A systematic review and meta-analyses. *American Journal of Psychiatry*, 173(6), 575–587. http://doi.org/10.1176/appi.ajp.2016.15091228

Mayo Clinic. (2013). *Drugs and Supplements: S. John's wort (Hypericum perforatum)*. Retrieved September 3, 2017 from: http://www.mayoclinic.org/drugs-supplements/st-johns-wort/evidence/hrb-20060053

Mannel, M. (2004). Drug Interactions with St John's Wort. *Drug Safety*, 27(11), 773–797. http://doi.org/10.2165/00002018-200427110-00003

Linde, K., Berner, M., Egger, M., & Mulrow, C. (2005). St John's wort for depression: Meta-analysis of randomised controlled trials. *British Journal of Psychiatry*, (186), 99–107. http://doi.org/10.1192/bjp.186.2.99

Saravanan, S., Srikumar, R., Manikandan, S., Jeya Parthasarathy, N., & Sheela Devi, R. (2007). Hypolipidemic effect of triphala in experimentally induced hypercholesteremic rats. *Yakugaku Zasshi : Journal of the Pharmaceutical Society of Japan*, 127(2), 385–388. http://doi.org/10.1248/yakushi.127.385

Baliga, M. S., Meera, S., Mathai, B., Rai, M. P., Pawar, V., & Palatty, P. L. (2012). Scientific validation of the ethnomedicinal properties of the Ayurvedic drug Triphala: A review. *Chinese Journal of Integrative Medicine*, 18(12), 946–954. http://doi.org/10.1007/s11655-012-1299-x

Motterli, R., Foresti, R., Bassi, R., & Green, C. J. (2000). CURCUMIN, AN ANTIOXIDANT AND ANTI-INFLAMMATORY AGENT, INDUCES HEME OXYGENASE-1 AND PROTECTS ENDOTHELIAL CELLS AGAINST OXIDATIVE STRESS. *Free Radical Biology and Medicine*, 28(8), 1303–1312.

Mishra, S., & Palanivelu, K. (2008). The effect of curcumin

(turmeric) on *Alzheimer's disease* : An overview. *Annals of Indian Academy of Neurology, 11*(1), 13. http://doi.org/10.4103/0972-2327.40220

Chattopadhyay, I., Biswas, K., Bandyopadhyay, U., & Banerjee, R. K. (2004). Turmeric and curcumin: Biological actions and medicinal applications. *Current Science, 87*(1), 44–53. http://doi.org/10.1248/bpb.29.1476

Tesch, B. J. (2003). Herbs commonly used by women: An evidence-based review. *American Journal of Obstetrics and Gynecology, 188*(5), S44–S55. http://doi.org/10.1016/S0011-5029(02)90011-8

Bent, S., Padula, A., Moore, D., Patterson, M., & Mehling, W. (2006). Valerian for Sleep: A Systematic Review and Meta-Analysis. *American Journal of Medicine.* http://doi.org/10.1016/j.amjmed.2006.02.026

Miyasaka, L. S., Atallah, Á. N., & Soares, B. (2006). Valerian for anxiety disorders. *Cochrane Database of Systematic Reviews,* (4). http://doi.org/10.1002/14651858.CD004515.pub2

Murti, K., Kaushik, M., Sangwan, Y., & Kaushik, A. (2011). Pharmacological Properties of Valeriana Officinalis-a Review. *Pharmacologyonline,* 3, 641–646. Retrieved from http://pharmacologyonline.silae.it/files/newsletter/2011/vol3/059.murti.pdf

Sarris, J., Panossian, A., Schweitzer, I., Stough, C., & Scholey, A. (2011). Herbal medicine for depression, anxiety and insomnia: A review of psychopharmacology and clinical evidence. *European Neuropsychopharmacology, 21*(12), 841–860. http://doi.org/10.1016/j.euroneuro.2011.04.002

Gromball, J., Beschorner, F., Wantzen, C., Paulsen, U., & Burkart, M. (2014). Hyperactivity, concentration difficulties and impulsiveness improve during seven weeks' treatment with valerian root and lemon balm extracts in primary school children. *Phytomedicine, 21*(8–9), 1098–1103. http://doi.org/10.1016/j.phymed.2014.04.004

Mirabi, P., Dolatian, M., Mojab, F., & Majd, H. A. (2011). Effects of valerian on the severity and systemic manifestations of dysmenorrhea. *International Journal of Gynecology and Obstetrics, 115*(3), 285–288. http://doi.org/10.1016/j.ijgo.2011.06.022

Sierpina, V. S., & Carter, R. (2002). Alternative and integrative treatment of fibromyalgia and chronic fatigue syndrome. *Clinics in Family Practice, 4*(4), 853–872. http://doi.org/10.1016/S1522-5720(02)00046-6

Spargias, K., Alexopoulos, E., Kyrzopoulos, S., Iacovis, P., Greenwood, D. C., Manginas, A., … Cokkinos, D. V. (2004). Ascorbic acid prevents contrast-mediated nephropathy in patients with renal dysfunction undergoing coronary angiography or intervention. *Circulation, 110*(18), 2837–2842. http://doi.org/10.1161/01.CIR.0000146396.19081.73

Simon, J. A. (1992). Vitamin C and cardiovascular disease: a review. *Journal of the American College of Nutrition, 11*(2), 107–125. Retrieved from http://europepmc.org/abstract/MED/1578086

Brody, S., Preut, R., Schommer, K., & Schürmeyer, T. H. (2002). A randomized controlled trial of high dose ascorbic acid for reduction of blood pressure, cortisol, and subjective responses to psychological stress. *Psychopharmacology, 159*(3), 319–324. http://doi.org/10.1007/s00213-001-0929-6

Anglin, R. E. S., Samaan, Z., Walter, S. D., & McDonald, S. D. (2013). Vitamin D deficiency and depression in adults: systematic review and meta-analysis. *The British Journal of Psychiatry, 202*(2), 100–107. http://doi.org/10.1192/bjp.bp.111.106666

Jorde, R., Sneve, M., Figenschau, Y., Svartberg, J., & Waterloo, K. (2008). Effects of vitamin D supplementation on symptoms of depression in overweight and obese subjects: Randomized double blind trial. *Journal of Internal Medicine, 264*(6), 599–609. http://doi.org/10.1111/j.1365-2796.2008.02008.x

Stroud, M. L., Stilgoe, S., Stott, V. E., Alhabian, O., & Salman, K. (2008). Vitamin D: A review. *Australian Family Physician, 37*(12), 1002–1005.

Mitri, J., Muraru, & Pittas, A. (2011). Vitamin D and type 2 diabetes: a systematic review. *European Journal of Clinical Nutrition, 65*(9), 1005–1015. http://doi.org/10.1038/ejcn.2011.118.Vitamin

Nachbar, F., & Korting, H. C. (1995). The role of vitamin E in normal and damaged skin. *Journal of Molecular Medicine, 73*(1), 7–17. http://doi.org/10.1007/BF00203614

Mills, S., & Bone, K. (2000). *Principles and practice of phytotherapy. Modern herbal medicine.* Churchill Livingstone.

Buvat, J., Siame-Mourot, C., Fourlinnie, J. C., Lemaire, A.,

Buvat-Herbaut, M., & Hermand, E. (1982). Androgens and prolactin levels in hirsute women with either polycystic ovaries or "borderline ovaries." *Fertility and Sterility*, 38(6), 695–700. http://doi.org/http://dx.doi.org/10.1016/S0015-0282(16)46696-7

Eltbogen, R., Litschgi, M., Gasser, U., Nebel, S., & Zahner, C. (2014). Vitex Agnus-Castus extract (Ze 440) improves symptoms in women with menstrual cycle irregularities. *Planta Med*, 80(16), SL19. http://doi.org/10.1055/s-0034-1394507

Grønli, O., Kvamme, J. M., Friborg, O., & Wynn, R. (2013). Zinc deficiency is common in several psychiatric disorders. *PLoS ONE*, 8(12), 6–12. http://doi.org/10.1371/journal.pone.0082793

Prasad, A.S. (2000). Effects of zinc deficiency on immune functions. *The Journal of Trace Elements in Experimental Medicine*, 13(1), 1–20. http://doi.org/10.1002/(SICI)1520-670X(2000)13:1<1::AID-JTRA3>3.0.CO;2-2

Prasad, A.S. (2009). Zinc: role in immunity, oxidative stress and chronic inflammation. *Current Opinion in Clinical Nutrition and Metabolic Care*, 12(6), 646–652. http://doi.org/10.1097/MCO.0b013e3283312956

Black, M. M. (1998). Zinc deficiency and child development. *The American Journal of Clinical Nutrition*, 68(2 Suppl), 464S–469S. http://doi.org/10.1016/j.bbi.2008.05.010

Liu, J., & Wuerker, A. (2005). Biosocial bases of aggressive and violent behavior–Implications for nursing studies. *International Journal of Nursing Studies*, 42(2), 229–241. http://doi.org/10.1016/j.ijnurstu.2004.06.007

Chapter 12: Getting Proactive

Pearlin, L. I., & Schooler, C. (1978). The structure of coping. Journal of Health and Social Behavior, 19(1), 2–21. http://doi.org/10.2307/2136539

Brady, C., Mousa, S. S., & Mousa, S. A. (2009). Polycystic ovary syndrome and its impact on women's quality of life: More than just an endocrine disorder. Drug, Healthcare and Patient Safety, 1(1), 9–15.

Scheier, M. F., & Carver, C. S. (1992). Effects of optimism on psychological and physical well-being: Theoretical overview and empirical update. Cognitive Therapy and Research, 16(2), 201–228. http://doi.org/10.1007/BF01173489

Peter McWilliams. (n.d.). BrainyQuote.com. Retrieved June 11, 2017, from BrainyQuote.com Web site: https://www.brainyquote.com/quotes/quotes/p/petermcwil125917.html

Janssen, O. E., Mehlmauer, N., Hahn, S., Offner, A. H., & Gärtner, R. (2004). High prevalence of autoimmune thyroiditis in patients with polycystic ovary syndrome. European Journal of Endocrinology / European Federation of Endocrine Societies, 150(3), 363–9. http://doi.org/10.1530/eje.0.1500363

Talbott, E., Guzick, D., Clerici, A., Berga, S., Detre, K., Weimer, K., & Kuller, L. (1995). Coronary Heart Disease Risk Factors in Women With Polycystic Ovary Syndrome. Arteriosclerosis, Thrombosis, and Vascular Biology, 15(7), 821 LP-826. Retrieved from http://atvb.ahajournals.org/content/15/7/821.abstract

Kabat-Zinn, J. (1994). Wherever you go, there you are: Mindfulness meditation in everyday life. (p. 4). New York: Hyperion.

Hofmann, S. G., Sawyer, A. T., Witt, A., & Oh, D. (2010). The effect of mindfulness-based therapy on anxiety and depression: A meta-analytic review. Journal of Consulting and Clinical Psychology, 78(2), 169–83. http://doi.org/10.1037/a0018555

Fox, K. C. R., Nijeboer, S., Dixon, M. L., Floman, J. L., Ellamil, M., Rumak, S. P., ... Christoff, K. (2014). Is meditation associated with altered brain structure? A systematic review and meta-analysis of morphometric neuroimaging in meditation practitioners. Neuroscience and Biobehavioral Reviews, 43, 48–73. http://doi.org/10.1016/j.neubiorev.2014.03.016

Chapter 13: Practicing Acceptance

Kamangar, F., Okhovat, J.-P., Schmidt, T., Beshay, A., Pasch, L., Cedars, M. I., ... Shinkai, K. (2015). Polycystic Ovary Syndrome: Special Diagnostic and Therapeutic Considerations for Children. Pediatric Dermatology, 32(5), 571–8. http://doi.org/10.1111/pde.12566

Chapter 15: Dealing With Pain

Soyupek, F., Yildiz, S., Akkus, S., Guney, M., Mungan, M. T., & Eris, S. (2010). The Frequency of Fibromyalgia Syndrome in Patients with Polycystic Ovary Syndrome. Journal of Musculoskeletal Pain, 18(2), 120–126. http://doi.org/10.3109/10582452.2010.483968

Banks, S. M., & Kerns, R. D. (1996). Explaining high rates of depression in chronic pain: A diathesis-stress framework. Psychological Bulletin, 119(1), 95–110. http://doi.org/10.1037/0033-2909.119.1.95

Dickerson, L. M., Mazyck, P. J., & Hunter, M. H. (2003). Premenstrual syndrome. American Family Physician, 67(8), 1743–1752. Retrieved from http://europepmc.org/abstract/MED/12725453

Azziz, R., Carmina, E., Dewailly, D., Diamanti-Kandarakis, E., Escobar-Morreale, H. F., Futterweit, W., ... Witchel, S. F. (2009). The Androgen Excess and PCOS Society criteria for the polycystic ovary syndrome: the complete task force report. Fertility and Sterility (Vol. 91). http://doi.org/10.1016/j.fertnstert.2008.06.035

McWilliams, L. A., Cox, B. J., & Enns, M. W. (2003). Mood and anxiety disorders associated with chronic pain: an examination in a nationally representative sample. Pain, 106(1–2), 127–133. http://doi.org/https://doi.org/10.1016/S0304-3959(03)00301-4

Chiesa, A., & Serretti, A. (2011). Mindfulness-Based Interventions for Chronic Pain: A Systematic Review of the Evidence. The Journal of Alternative and Complementary Medicine, 17(1), 83–93. http://doi.org/10.1089/acm.2009.0546

Appendix: Prescription Medications

Rao, T. S. S., Asha, M. R., Ramesh, B. N., & Rao, K. S. J. (2008). Understanding nutrition, depression and mental illnesses. *Indian Journal of Psychiatry*, 50(2), 77–82. http://doi.org/10.4103/0019-5545.42391

Araujo, O. E., & Flowers, F. P. (1984). Stevens-Johnson syndrome. *The Journal of Emergency Medicine*, 2(2), 129–135. http://doi.org/http://dx.doi.org/10.1016/0736-4679(84)90332-9

De Maat, S., Dekker, J., Schoevers, R., & De Jonghe, F. (2006). Relative efficacy of psychotherapy and pharmacotherapy in the treatment of depression: A meta-analysis. *Psychotherapy Research, 16*(August 2015), 566–578. http://doi.org/10.1080/10503300600756402

Hill, K. P. (2015). Medical Marijuana for Treatment of Chronic Pain and Other Medical and Psychiatric Problems. *Jama, 313*(24), 2474. http://doi.org/10.1001/jama.2015.6199

Klein, T. W. (2005). Cannabinoid-based drugs as anti-inflammatory therapeutics. *Nature Reviews Immunology, 5*(5), 400–411. http://doi.org/10.1038/nri1602

Tramèr, M. R., Carroll, D., Campbell, F. A., Reynolds, D. J., Moore, R. A., & McQuay, H. J. (2001). Cannabinoids for control of chemotherapy induced nausea and vomiting: quantitative systematic review. *BMJ (Clinical Research Ed.), 323*(7303), 16–21. http://doi.org/10.1136/bmj.323.7303.16

Lynch, M. E., & Campbell, F. (2011). Cannabinoids for treatment of chronic non-cancer pain; a systematic review of randomized trials. *British Journal of Clinical Pharmacology, 72*(5), 735–744. http://doi.org/10.1111/j.1365-2125.2011.03970.x

Bergamaschi, M. M., Queiroz, R. H. C., Chagas, M. H. N., de Oliveira, D. C. G., De Martinis, B. S., Kapczinski, F., ... Crippa, J. A. S. (2011). Cannabidiol reduces the anxiety induced by simulated public speaking in treatment-naïve social phobia patients.

Maa, E., & Figi, P. (2014). The case for medical marijuana in epilepsy. *Epilepsia, 55*(6), 783–786. http://doi.org/10.1111/epi.12610

Campos, A. C., Fogaça, M. V., Sonego, A. B., & Guimarães, F. S. (2016). Cannabidiol, neuroprotection and neuropsychiatric disorders. *Pharmacological Research, 112*(June), 119–127. http://doi.org/10.1016/j.phrs.2016.01.033

Katalinic, N., Lai, R., Somogyi, A., Mitchell, P. B., Glue, P., & Loo, C. K. (2013). Ketamine as a new treatment for depression: a review of its efficacy and adverse effects. *The Australian and New Zealand Journal of Psychiatry, 47*(8), 710–27. http://doi.org/10.1177/0004867413486842

Hudetz, J. A., & Pagel, P. S. (2010). Neuroprotection by Ketamine: A Review of the Experimental and Clinical Evidence. *Journal of*

Cardiothoracic and Vascular Anesthesia, 24(1), 131–142. http://doi.org/10.1053/j.jvca.2009.05.008

Lefaucheur, J. P., Andre-Obadia, N., Antal, A., Ayache, S. S., Baeken, C., Benninger, D. H., ... Garcia-Larrea, L. (2014). Evidence-based guidelines on the therapeutic use of repetitive transcranial magnetic stimulation (rTMS). *Clin Neurophysiol, 125*(11), 2150–2206. http://doi.org/S1388-2457(14)00296-X [pii]\r10.1016/j.clinph.2014.05.021 [doi]

Lam, R. W., Chan, P., Wilkins-Ho, M., & Yatham, L. N. (2008). Repetitive transcranial magnetic stimulation for treatment-resistant depression: a systematic review and metaanalysis. *Canadian Journal of Psychiatry. Revue Canadienne de Psychiatrie, 53*(9), 621–631. Retrieved from http://ovidsp.ovid.com/ovidweb.cgi?T=JS&PAGE=reference&D=med5&NEWS=N&AN=18801225

Insel, T. (December 6, 2011). Antidepressants: A complicated picture. *National Institute of Mental Health.* Retrieved 8/13/17 from: https://www.nimh.nih.gov/about/directors/thomas-insel/blog/2011/antidepressants-a-complicated-picture.shtml

Pagnin, D., de Queiroz, V., Pini, S., & Cassano, G. B. (2004). Efficacy of ECT in Depression: A Meta-Analytic Review. *The Journal of ECT, 20*(1), 13–20. http://doi.org/10.1097/00124509-200403000-00004

Kellner, C. H., Fink, M., Knapp, R., Petrides, G., Husain, M., Rummans, T., ... Malur, C. (2005). Relief of Expressed Suicidal Intent by ECT: A Consortium for Research in ECT Study. *American Journal of Psychiatry, 162*(5), 977–982. http://doi.org/10.1176/appi.ajp.162.5.977.Relief

Caroff, S. N., Ungvari, G. S., Bhati, M. T., Datto, C. J., & O'Reardon, J. P. (2007). Catatonia and Prediction of Response to Electroconvulsive Therapy. *Psychiatric Annals, 37*(1), 57–65.

Lisanby, S. H. (2007). Electroconvulsive Therapy for Depression. *The New England Journal of Medicine, 19357*(8), 1939–45. http://doi.org/10.1056/NEJMct075234

Moore, E. M., Mander, A. G., Ames, D., Kotowicz, M. A., Carne, R. P., Brodaty, H., ... Watters, D. A. (2013). Increased risk of cognitive impairment in patients with diabetes is associated with metformin. *Diabetes Care, 36*(10), 2981–2987. http://doi.org/10.2337/dc13-0229

Shaheen, N., & Ransohoff, D. F. (2002). Gastroesophageal Reflux,

Barrett Esophagus, and Esophageal Cancer. *JAMA, 287*(15), 1972. http://doi.org/10.1001/jama.287.15.1972

Vélez, L. M., & Motta, A. B. (2014). Association between polycystic ovary syndrome and metabolic syndrome. *Current Medicinal Chemistry, 21*(35), 3999–4012. http://doi.org/10.2174/09298673216661409151410 30

Alpert, J. E., & Fava, M. (1997). Nutrition and depression: the role of folate. *Nutrition Reviews, 55*(5), 145–149. http://doi.org/10.1111/j.1753-4887.1997.tb06468.x

Umbreit, J. (2005). Iron deficiency: A concise review. *American Journal of Hematology, 78*(3), 225–231. http://doi.org/10.1002/ajh.20249

Goebels, N., & Soyka, M. (2000). Dementia Associated With Vitamin B 12 Deficiency: Presentation of Two Cases and Review of the Literature. *The Journal of Neuropsychiatry and Clinical Neurosciences, 123*(12), 389–394. http://doi.org/10.1176/appi.neuropsych.12.3.389

Rasmussen, H. H., Mortensen, P. B., & Jensen, I. W. (1990). Depression and Magnesium Deficiency. *The International Journal of Psychiatry in Medicine, 19*(1), 57–63. http://doi.org/10.2190/NKCD-1RB1-QMA9-G1VN

Hollick, M. (2007). Vitamin D Deficiency. *The New England Journal of Medicine, 357,* 266–281. http://doi.org/10.1016/j.mam.2008.05.004

Verbeek, D. E. P., van Riezen, J., de Boer, R. A., van Melle, J. P., & de Jonge, P. (2011). A Review on the Putative Association Between Beta-Blockers and Depression. *Heart Failure Clinics, 7*(1), 89–99. http://doi.org/http://dx.doi.org/10.1016/j.hfc.2010.08.006

Talbott, E., Guzick, D., Clerici, A., Berga, S., Detre, K., Weimer, K., & Kuller, L. (1995). Coronary Heart Disease Risk Factors in Women With Polycystic Ovary Syndrome. *Arteriosclerosis, Thrombosis, and Vascular Biology, 15*(7), 821 LP-826. Retrieved from http://atvb.ahajournals.org/content/15/7/821.abstract

Bays, H. (2006). Statin Safety: An Overview and Assessment of the Data—2005. *The American Journal of Cardiology, 97*(8), S6–S26. http://doi.org/http://dx.doi.org/10.1016/j.amjcard.2005.12.006

Wagstaff, L. R., Mitton, M. W., Arvik, B. M., & Doraiswamy, P. M. (2003). Statin-Associated Memory Loss: Analysis of 60 Case Reports and Review of the Literature. *Pharmacotherapy: The Journal of Human*

Pharmacology and Drug Therapy, 23(7), 871–880. http://doi.org/10.1592/phco.23.7.871.32720

Janssen, O. E., Mehlmauer, N., Hahn, S., Offner, A. H., & Gärtner, R. (2004). High prevalence of autoimmune thyroiditis in patients with polycystic ovary syndrome. *European Journal of Endocrinology / European Federation of Endocrine Societies, 150*(3), 363–9. http://doi.org/10.1530/eje.0.1500363

Ladenson, P. W., Singer, P. a, Ain, K. B., Bagchi, N., Bigos, S. T., Levy, E. G., … Cohen, H. D. (2000). American Thyroid Association Guidelines for Detection of Thyroid Dysfunction. *Archives of Internal Medicine, 160*(July), 1573–1575. http://doi.org/10.1001/archinte.160.11.157

Sansone, R. A., & Sansone, L. A. (2011). Allergic rhinitis: Relationships with anxiety and mood syndromes. *Innovations in Clinical Neuroscience, 8*(7), 12–17. http://doi.org/10.1007/978-0-387-49979-6_21

Zierau, L., Gade, E. J., Lindenberg, S., Backer, V., & Thomsen, S. F. (2016). Coexistence of asthma and polycystic ovary syndrome: A concise review. *Respiratory Medicine, 119*, 155–159. http://doi.org/http://dx.doi.org/10.1016/j.rmed.2016.08.025

Printed in the United States
By Bookmasters